CSIRO
PROTEIN PLUS

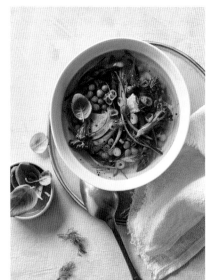
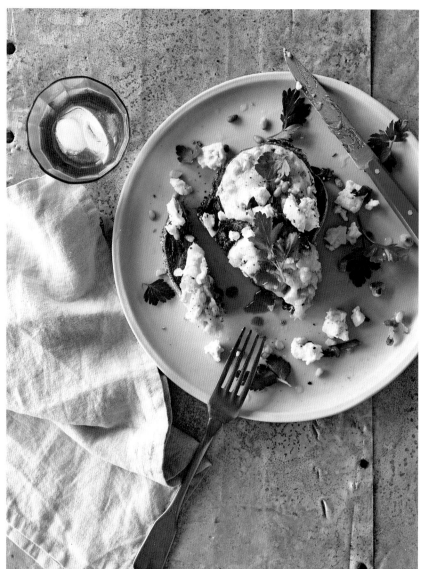
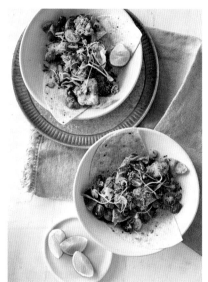
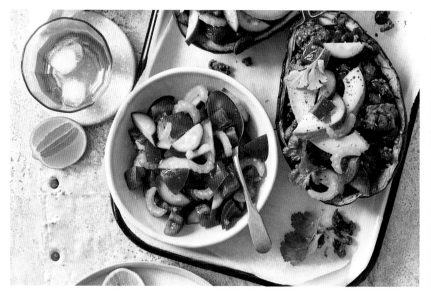
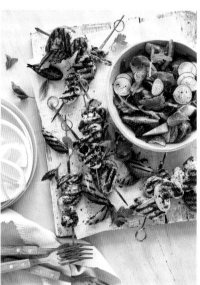

CSIRO
PROTEIN PLUS
NUTRITION AND EXERCISE PLAN

**Dr Jane Bowen, Professor Grant Brinkworth
and Genevieve James-Martin**

Photography by Rob Palmer

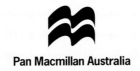

Pan Macmillan Australia

Contents

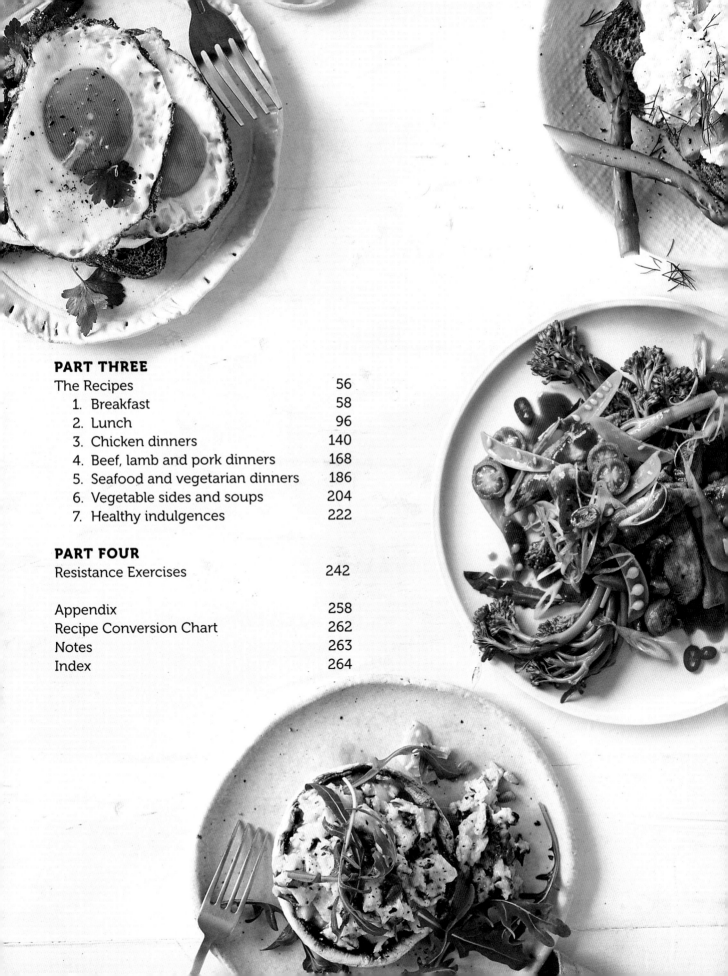

Introduction

CSIRO is at the forefront of nutritional science and lifestyle research in Australia. We also have a track record of translating these scientific findings into a variety of practical and easy-to-follow diet and exercise programs that Australians can use to improve their health. As the science evolves, so too does the information we provide to the community.

In 2005, we published *The CSIRO Total Wellbeing Diet*. This book sold over 1 million copies and went on to become Australia's bestselling diet and lifestyle plan. Focusing on weight loss, it advocates a higher protein, low-fat, wholefood dietary pattern with a moderate amount of low-GI carbohydrates. This message has become the basis for a number of books and a successful interactive online weightloss program, totalwellbeingdiet.com.

The central principle of a higher protein dietary approach was also applied to improving heart health and reducing the risk of diabetes in *The CSIRO Healthy Heart Program* and *The CSIRO and Baker IDI Diabetes Diet and Lifestyle Plan* respectively.

The CSIRO Low-carb Diet was based on further research we conducted on the short- and long-term effects of a lower carbohydrate intake and higher intakes of healthy (unsaturated) fat than recommended previously. This low-carb diet plan can achieve excellent weight loss results and is highly effective in stabilising blood glucose and reducing the need for diabetes medications.

This book, *CSIRO Protein Plus Nutrition and Exercise Plan*, is our latest contribution to the conversation on health through nutrition and physical activity. Here we present brand new research from both CSIRO and other trusted science bodies around the world on the benefits of spreading protein consumption across the day, and the combination of higher dietary protein and resistance exercise.

Based on this emerging research, the four key take-home points are:

* A higher amount of dietary protein than current national dietary guidelines recommend may be required for optimum health for many adults.
* Evenly spreading dietary protein across breakfast, lunch and dinner may provide additional benefits. Typically, Australians eat little protein at breakfast, and most at dinnertime.
* Combining regular resistance exercise with eating adequate dietary protein can increase the amount of muscle mass relative to body fat.
* Animal- and plant-based protein foods provide different nutrients, and are digested and absorbed by the body differently. These are important considerations for meeting protein needs.

This book summarises the latest science about why and how we include protein in our diet – in terms of quantity, dietary sources and when it is eaten. We believe this information will be of great benefit across the community because dietary protein is essential to good health at all stages of life. We also identify some specific benefits that will be of interest to many adults in the community:

1. **Weight management.** Protein helps manage appetite, reduce food cravings and boost metabolism.

2. **Improved physical function, strength and health.** Adequate dietary protein, combined with regular resistance exercise, helps build and maintain lean body mass and strength. This can lower the risk of diabetes, heart disease, some cancers and osteoarthritis.
3. **Healthy ageing.** Adequate dietary protein, combined with resistance exercise, helps preserve muscle function as we age, in turn maintaining strength, reducing the likelihood of injuries and supporting active and independent lives.

Weight management is a key component of much of the protein research that has been conducted by CSIRO and other laboratories around the world. With around two-thirds of Australian adults being either overweight or obese, weight management is an important matter. However, this book is *not* a diet book as such (which typically includes structured meal plans for a defined period that are tailored to different energy requirements). Instead, this book focuses on the multiple health benefits of following a long-term, balanced and nutritious eating pattern that features dietary protein in adequate amounts, distributed more evenly across breakfast, lunch and dinner, along with regular resistance exercise.

Australians are consuming too many foods that are high in saturated fat, sugar, salt and alcohol, and low in beneficial nutrients. What's more, about 23% of our dietary protein comes from these 'discretionary' foods. This book will help readers shift towards more nutritious protein foods, along with improving overall diet quality by having core foods – such as vegetables, wholegrains, dairy, meat and alternatives, fruit and healthy fats – at the heart of the eating plan.

Part One of this book provides a summary of the role of dietary protein in our bodies, its different sources and their qualities, with an update on the science regarding the benefits of a higher protein intake and a more even distribution across the day.

In **Part Two** we provide specific information on high protein foods and sample meal plans to show how a more even daily dietary protein distribution can be achieved in a balanced, healthy diet. For people who are particularly interested in more detailed dietary support for weight loss, *The CSIRO Total Wellbeing Diet* is a 12-week program with easy online tools and Protein Balance meal plans tailored to your energy needs (totalwellbeingdiet.com).

Part Three is a treasure trove of higher protein recipes for breakfast, lunch and dinner. Delicious, simple and nutritionally balanced, these recipes feature plenty of vegetables and salads (and so are rich in fibre), use healthy fats and some wholegrain, low-GI carbohydrates, while keeping levels of refined sugars, salt and saturated fats low.

Part Four provides readers with a program of simple, home-based exercises that can be easily incorporated into your daily routine.

As always, CSIRO remains committed to providing Australians with the best possible dietary advice based on the very latest research. *CSIRO Protein Plus Nutrition and Exercise Plan* **is an important next chapter in the protein story, showing Australians how to best use this essential nutrient for optimum health benefits.**

About the authors

Dr Jane Bowen

Jane is a senior research scientist and dietitian at CSIRO. She completed her PhD studying the role of dietary protein on appetite regulation and weight management. Her food and nutrition research focuses on achieving optimal metabolic health outcomes through diet and weight management. She is committed to applying research findings to practical information and programs that support people to lead healthy lifestyles. This work has spanned contributing to *The CSIRO Total Wellbeing Diet* books, developing meal replacement weight-loss programs, authoring *The CSIRO Wellbeing Plan for Kids*, coordinating the 2007 Australian Children's National Nutrition and Physical Activity Survey and exploring opportunities to minimise food waste. As a food lover and mum to three young children, Jane is motivated to share trustworthy and no-nonsense food and dietary advice that the Australian community can use in their everyday lives.

Professor Grant Brinkworth

Grant is a senior principal research scientist in Clinical Nutrition and Exercise Science at CSIRO Health and Biosecurity. He has a PhD and expertise in diet, nutrition and exercise science. Grant has more than 18 years' experience leading large-scale, multi-disciplinary clinical research teams and studies evaluating the effects of dietary patterns, foods, nutritional components and physical exercise on weight loss, metabolic disease risk management, health and performance. Grant has particular interests in developing effective lifestyle solutions for achieving optimal weight, metabolic health and diabetes management, and understanding the role of higher protein, lower-carbohydrate dietary patterns for health management. He has published more than 80 peer-reviewed research papers on the topic of diet and lifestyle management of obesity and related diseases and was co-author of the bestselling book *The CSIRO Low-carb Diet*.

Genevieve James-Martin

Genevieve is a research dietitian at CSIRO. She has developed and delivered dietary interventions for numerous clinical trials to explore the link between foods, diets and nutrients, and health. Her work has also focused on translating research outcomes into public health services and commercial programs that assist Australians in making healthier dietary choices. This has included digital tools to boost vegetable consumption and developing healthy menu guidelines for restaurants. Genevieve thrives on turning her understanding of good nutrition into delicious meals and believes healthy eating should be simple, practical and, above all, tasty.

Acknowledgements

We would like to sincerely thank the numerous colleagues, collaborators and reviewers who have provided guidance and feedback throughout the preparation of this book. From CSIRO we thank Dr Gilly Hendrie, Dr Rob Grenfell, Ofa Fitzgibbons, Asaesja Young, Dr Beverly Mühlhäusler, Dr Brad Ridoutt and Dr Atul Kacker. Thanks also to Professor Stuart Phillips, Director of Physical Activity Centre of Excellence at McMaster University (Canada), Associate Professor Heather Leidy of University of Texas, Austin (USA), and Distinguished Professor Paul Moughan, Riddet Institute Fellow Laureate at Massey University (NZ), who provided their professional expertise in reviewing and advising on the book's content.

Special thanks go to Professor Manny Noakes (previously the Nutrition and Health Research Director at CSIRO Health and Biosecurity), who initiated the vision for this book and provided substantial content and professional guidance throughout its development. Professor Noakes is a world-leading expert in the role of dietary protein and nutrition for weight management and promoting health and wellbeing, and her expert guidance, scientific ideas and mentorship over many years has been invaluable.

Furthermore, this book and the concepts communicated within it are underpinned not only by the clinical research undertaken at CSIRO over the years, but also by the scientific knowledge and research driven and produced by many other world-class researchers around the world. We would like to recognise the enormous efforts of the many scientific research leaders and groups who have conducted high-quality research, which continues to advance concepts in understanding the role of dietary protein and how it can promote health and sustainability in our communities.

We would also like to acknowledge the hard work of the editorial and publishing team at Pan Macmillan Australia. To Ingrid Ohlsson, for her unwavering enthusiasm and passion for improving the health and wellbeing of our communities through better diet, nutrition and lifestyle; to Virginia Birch, Katri Hilden, Rachel Carter, Naomi van Groll and Sally Devenish for their tireless work and support throughout the editorial and production process; and to publicist Lucy Inglis for her ongoing commitment and dedication. Thanks to Tracey Pattison for her beautifully crafted and mouthwatering recipes, to Sarah Odgers for her wonderful design, and to Peta Dent, Sarah-Jane Hallett, Emma Knowles and Rob Palmer for bringing the recipes to life with the food photography. Thanks also to our exercise models Victoria Stilwell and Evan Stilwell.

Finally, a big thank you to the volunteers who have participated in the numerous research trials we have conducted over the years. Without their dedication, we would not be able to continue to advance our understanding of protein science and its range of health impacts.

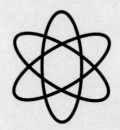

PART ONE

The Power of Protein

The role of proteins

Often described as the 'building blocks' of the body, proteins are large, complex molecules that have many diverse roles in our body, all of which are essential for life.

Proteins do most of the work in our cells, and play a key role in how our organs function. Our bodies use protein to build, maintain, repair and replace tissues. Our muscles are made of protein, and our other tissues contain a protein called collagen, which acts like a glue to connect and support our muscles, bones, tendons, ligaments, cartilage, blood vessels, organs and even our skin.

Some of our hormones are proteins, and our food is digested by enzymes, which are also proteins. Our immune system produces proteins called antibodies to fight bacterial infections. Oxygen is transported through our bloodstream by the protein haemoglobin.

Our body can make, or 'synthesise', all of these different proteins. But to do this, it needs to be supplied with all the necessary ingredients, in the form of dietary protein from the foods we eat. Dietary proteins are found in both animal and plant foods.

Here are some of the roles proteins play in our body:

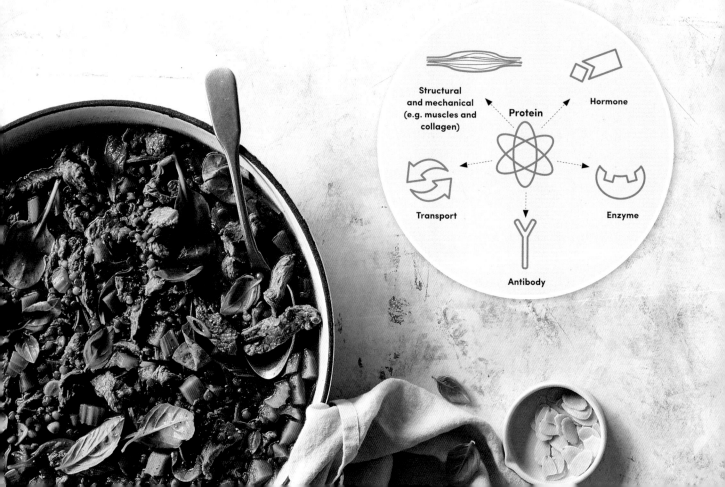

Structural and mechanical (e.g. muscles and collagen)

Hormone

Protein

Transport

Enzyme

Antibody

Dietary proteins

All proteins are made up of long chains of amino acids, which twist into 3D shapes. Each protein has a unique shape that gives it a distinct function — similar to the way in which the shape of a key will fit just one lock. The 'recipe' for each protein is coded in our DNA.

There are 20 different amino acids, and our body combines them in unique ways to make all the proteins we need to survive. Of these 20 amino acids, our bodies can make 11, and so we call these non-essential (these are alanine, arginine, asparagine, aspartate, cysteine, glutamate, glutamine, glycine, proline, serine and tyrosine). The other nine are called essential amino acids, because it's **essential** that we get them through the food that we eat. These are histidine, isoleucine, leucine, lysine, methionine, phenylalanine, threonine, tryptophan and valine.

Not all dietary proteins are alike

The dietary proteins we eat are digested by enzymes, called proteases, into short strings of amino acids (peptides) and single amino acids. This process begins in the stomach and continues in the small intestine, where amino acids are absorbed into the circulation and are then used for protein synthesis (making new proteins). The 'quality' of the protein in different foods depends on:

1. whether or not it contains any/all of the nine essential amino acids our body needs to synthesise new proteins, and
2. the relative ease of digestibility in the stomach and small intestine, along with its absorption — in other words, how much of the protein consumed is actually taken up into the body.

Dietary proteins that come from animal sources (for example, meat, dairy foods and eggs) are considered high quality because they contain all nine essential amino acids in high amounts, and they are more readily digested, absorbed and used by the body. In addition to being protein-rich, they are also nutrient-dense; collectively they provide a good source of iron, zinc, omega-3 fats, vitamin B12 and calcium.

Most vegetable proteins (apart from soy protein) are considered lower quality because they lack one or more of the essential amino acids. Plant proteins are also **less efficiently absorbed by our gut**. This is because they typically contain a significant amount of dietary fibre and compounds, which can reduce the body's ability to access, digest and utilise the protein.

However, people who follow a vegetarian diet can generally meet their protein needs by choosing from a wide variety of protein-rich plant-based foods. You can read more about plant-based diets on page 26.

EMERGING PROTEIN SCIENCE:
Measuring protein quality

A new measure of protein quality called Digestible Indispensable Amino Acid Score (DIAAS) has recently been developed by the Food and Agriculture Organization (FAO) of the United Nations. DIAAS is now the accepted method of assessing the quality of dietary protein. It takes into account individual essential amino acids, along with the extent to which the protein is digested and the amino acids become available to the body. A score is assigned which can be used to rank different protein foods. Only a few foods have had their DIAAS score calculated so far but, as this area of science grows, we can build our understanding of how to feed our growing global population sustainably using a variety of different plant and animal protein sources and achieving the most favourable health outcomes.

Rethinking dietary protein guidelines

How much dietary protein do we need?

Our body's requirement for dietary protein varies during the different stages of life. For example, protein needs are relatively higher during periods of childhood growth, and also during pregnancy and breastfeeding.

How much dietary protein you need also depends on **your weight**, as well as your age and sex. Recent evidence, supported by many eminent international research groups, shows that some adults may benefit from a daily protein intake higher than the current recommendations shown below.

Current Australian recommended dietary intakes (RDIs) for protein

(an average for healthy adults, based on an amount of protein for each kilogram of bodyweight, and also taking into account a person's sex and age)

For **healthy** adults aged **19–70 years**:

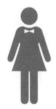

Women need:
0.75 grams
of protein per
kg per day

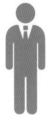

Men need:
0.84 grams
of protein per
kg per day

For **healthy** adults aged **70+ years**, this requirement increases by 25%:

Women need:
0.94 grams
of protein per
kg per day

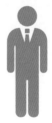

Men need:
1.07 grams
of protein per
kg per day

These recommendations were developed in 2006, based on research published prior to that time. Since then, a significant amount of high-quality research has been conducted. Based on these findings, a number of expert committees and scientific leaders in dietary protein from around the world have concluded that...

A higher protein intake, ranging between 1.2 grams and 1.6 grams per kilogram of bodyweight per day, is a more ideal target for achieving optimal health outcomes for most healthy adults.

This reference range can be used to calculate a daily dietary protein intake range. If your weight is above the healthy range, it is advisable to seek advice from an accredited practising dietitian to determine an optimal dietary protein intake to aim for.

Protein for building muscle mass

The current RDI for protein assumes individuals have adequate amounts of muscle mass. However, most Australians have low levels of physical activity, and consequently have a less than ideal amount of muscle mass. Additional dietary protein (and regular resistance exercise) is required for building muscle mass. To learn more, see pages 16–21.

Protein for weight loss

The current Australian RDI for dietary protein assumes that individuals are not trying to lose weight. However, people who are on a weight-loss program will benefit from higher amounts of dietary protein – and given that 60–70% of our adult population are overweight or obese and could benefit from reducing their weight, this applies to many of us. To learn more, see pages 22–23.

Protein for healthy ageing

It is an unfortunate fact of ageing that we lose both muscle mass and muscle strength as we get older. Since nearly one in six Australians are aged over 65, this affects many people in our community. New research is showing that a higher intake of high-quality dietary protein, along with resistance exercise, can help to minimise this decline in muscle. To learn more about these simple lifestyle strategies, see pages 24–25.

Protein for plant-based diets

The current Australian RDI for dietary protein is based on the assumption that mostly high-quality dietary proteins are consumed. However, most Australians consume a mix of animal- and plant-based proteins, along with a large amount of discretionary foods, which means we obtain only about half our protein from high-quality protein sources. Therefore, a higher amount of protein is advisable for people following vegetarian and vegan diets. To learn more about this, turn to pages 26–28.

Improving body composition with dietary protein

Body composition describes the relative amounts of the different tissues your body is composed of, distinguishing body fat from lean body mass.

Your **lean body mass** is the amount of body weight that isn't fat. It includes the weight of your muscles, skeleton and internal organs. Your **muscle mass** includes your **skeletal muscles** (the muscles surrounding your bones), your **smooth and cardiac muscles** (such as your heart and digestive muscles), and the water contained within these muscles. The amount of smooth muscle you have doesn't really change throughout life, but your skeletal muscle mass can. You can build your skeletal muscle mass through resistance exercise, or conversely lose some of it through inactivity and a sedentary lifestyle.

Why is body composition important?

Having a higher lean body mass and a healthy level of body fat is associated with better health, regardless of your age or stage of life. Studies show these are associated with a lower risk of:

* insulin resistance and type 2 diabetes
* cardiovascular disease
* certain cancers
* osteoarthritis
* sleep apnoea
* sexual dysfunction and infertility.

There are many reasons why maintaining a healthy amount of muscle mass is important for good health and wellbeing:

* Having higher muscle mass is associated with greater muscle strength, and a healthy body composition is associated with a reduced risk of heart disease, type 2 diabetes and all-cause mortality.
* Having more skeletal muscle is associated with better bone strength and health.
* A higher skeletal muscle mass helps burn fat, because it increases the amount of energy (kilojoules) your body uses. Just as a bigger car engine needs more fuel to keep it running, having more muscle mass means your body needs more energy to fuel your muscles. Having more muscle increases your basal metabolic rate, which means you burn more energy even while at rest, and this increase in the amount of kilojoules used can help to manage bodyweight.
* Our muscles help us engage in physical activity and live an active lifestyle. This is particularly important as we get older because it helps us perform the activities of daily living and stay independent.

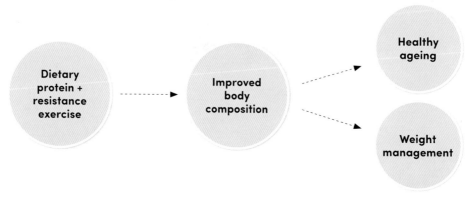

Dietary protein + resistance exercise → Improved body composition → Healthy ageing / Weight management

Unfortunately, most Australians lead very sedentary lifestyles, resulting in a lower proportion of skeletal muscle mass. Based on data from the Australian Bureau of Statistics, 60–70% of the population has low levels of physical activity.

Many people, in fact more than 60% of Australian adults, are also overweight (36%) or obese (28%). This combination of sedentary lifestyles and being overweight or obese means that the majority of people have a less than optimal overall body composition.

The good news from scientific studies is that combining a higher-protein diet with regular resistance exercise is an effective approach for people wishing to improve their body composition by reducing their fat mass level and increasing their lean body mass levels.

Boosting your muscle mass

Building and maintaining muscle mass has enormous benefits for general health and wellbeing across all stages of life. Whether you are young or older, are already a healthy weight or wanting to lose weight, research shows that **resistance exercise training** has many important health benefits.

Resistance exercise — also known as strength or weight training — is any form of exercise that requires your skeletal muscles to contract and generate force against resistance, such as bodyweight exercises, circuit training, pilates, lifting weights or using stretch bands. Undertaking regular resistance exercise leads to increases in muscle strength, endurance and tone.

What's more, combining **resistance exercise** with **adequate dietary protein** is a powerful combination for increasing muscle and reducing body fat.

To get started on your very own resistance exercise plan, see the simple but very effective home-based program we've devised on pages 242–257.

RESISTANCE
EXERCISE
+
DIETARY PROTEIN
=
**A DYNAMIC
DUO**

Studies have shown that resistance exercise:

* helps us build and maintain muscle mass
* increases our muscle function and strength
* improves our mobility
* increases our metabolic rate and promotes kilojoule burning
* improves our mood and general wellbeing, and reduces depressive symptoms
* reduces anxiety symptoms in healthy people, and those with a physical or mental illness
* improves sleep quality, and reduces the severity of sleep apnoea.

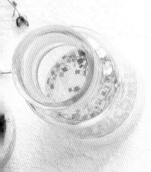
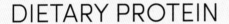
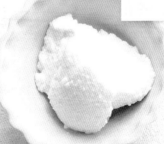
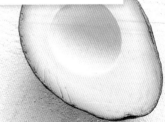

What happens to body composition during weight loss?

Most of us know all too well that when we consume more energy (kilojoules) than our body needs, we gain weight. Even though this may occur gradually, it also happens easily.

The reverse, of course, is also true: to lose weight, we need to consume fewer kilojoules than our body needs. However, we all know that losing weight isn't always quite as easy as this straightforward formula would suggest. Consuming fewer kilojoules than our body needs creates an 'energy deficit' — and during a prolonged energy deficit our body uses its energy stores to provide the extra energy we need to survive.

Most of this stored energy comes from breaking down body fat, but a smaller portion also comes from breaking down muscle mass. As we have just described, it is ideal to **maintain, not lose, muscle mass** as this keeps our basal metabolic rate higher.

At CSIRO, we have conducted many weight-loss studies investigating the optimal way to minimise the loss of lean mass and maximise fat loss when we lose weight. Our research, and other research conducted in leading laboratories around the world, consistently shows that energy-restricted diets that are higher in dietary protein help achieve this, particularly when combined with resistance exercise.

The combination of a resistance exercise program (such as the one in Part 4) with an energy-restricted, higher-protein eating plan can help you achieve weight loss while also maintaining your muscle mass.

BMI CLASSIFICATIONS

less than 18.49 = Underweight
18.5–24.9 = Normal weight
25.0–29.9 = Overweight
greater than 30 = Obese

Measuring your body composition

After all this information about muscle mass, you may be wondering about your own body composition, and how you could track changes over time.

The **body mass index** (BMI) classification is a convenient way to estimate body composition using your height and weight. It gives a reasonable indication of the amount of body fat you are likely to have, based on whether your BMI is classified as underweight, normal weight, overweight or obese.

Overweight and obese classifications are generally associated with higher body fatness, and this may increase the risk of numerous lifestyle-related diseases.

You can calculate your BMI by dividing your weight (in kg) by the square of your height (in metres).

BMI = weight in kilograms/ height (metres) × height (metres)

SAMPLE BMI CALCULATION

Mike weighs 105 kilograms and is 172 cm (1.72 metres) tall. **His BMI is therefore:**

105 kg / (1.72 m × 1.72 m) = 35.5

Mike is classified as obese, and this may indicate a high amount of body fat. Additional body composition measures can help determine this.

While BMI is very easy to measure, it is not an ideal tool for predicting your actual body composition. Your BMI can underestimate or overestimate your body fatness, because your relative amount of fat and lean body mass will also depend on your age, sex, ethnicity, body shape (as measured by your waist circumference), and the level and types of physical activity you regularly do. See page 258 for another way to measure your body composition, or if you'd prefer to use an online tool, visit totalwellbeingdiet.com/bmi-calculator.

Waist circumference

Measuring your waist circumference is another simple way to better understand your body composition. It gives an indication of the distribution of excess body fat around your middle (compared to your hips and thighs), which is a predictor of higher risk of diseases such as cardiovascular disease and diabetes.

To check your waist measurement:
1.. Feel for the top of your hip bone and the bottom of your ribs.
2. Wrap a tape measure around your waist, positioning it midway between the top of your hip bone and the bottom of your ribs.
3. Breathe out normally, then check your waist measurement.

Your health is at risk if your waist size is:

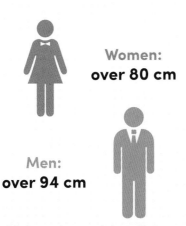

**Women:
over 80 cm**

**Men:
over 94 cm**

If you think you're at risk, talk to your doctor or accredited practising dietitian about what you can do.

Measuring lean mass

Thanks to advances in technology, bioelectric impedance analysis (BIA) scales are another way to measure your fat and lean body mass. Many scales on the market now come with BIA capabilities.

Bioelectric impedance analysis measures the level of opposition (or 'impedance') to the flow of an electric current through a person's body. Most lean mass has a high water content, and is highly conductive of an electric current, while fat has a lower water content and impedes the electrical flow. By combining the impedance measure with your height and weight, the BIA scale will estimate your body fat percentage, as well as your fat-free body mass (your lean mass, including water, organs and bone).

These devices are easy to use, and although they may not be as accurate as other techniques used in clinical research studies, they are useful for tracking progress if you're trying to change your body composition. It is important to be mindful that the accuracy of these devices can also be affected by your state of hydration, so it is best to use them at the same time of day and after emptying your bladder.

BIA scales are very safe to use regularly, although they are not recommended for anyone with an implanted electrical device, such as a pacemaker.

As yet, there are no agreed-upon optimal body composition targets to assess your BIA readings; however BIA scales can be used to monitor changes in your body composition over time.

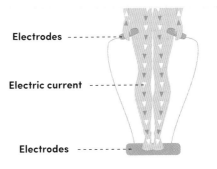

Electrodes ----------

Electric current ----------

Electrodes ----------

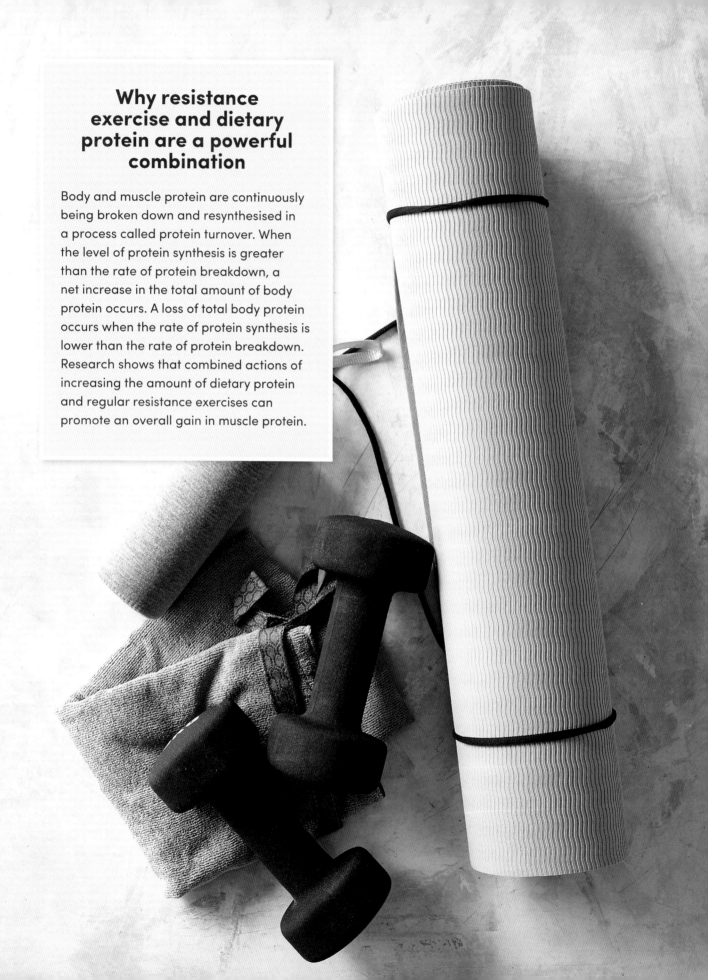

Why resistance exercise and dietary protein are a powerful combination

Body and muscle protein are continuously being broken down and resynthesised in a process called protein turnover. When the level of protein synthesis is greater than the rate of protein breakdown, a net increase in the total amount of body protein occurs. A loss of total body protein occurs when the rate of protein synthesis is lower than the rate of protein breakdown. Research shows that combined actions of increasing the amount of dietary protein and regular resistance exercises can promote an overall gain in muscle protein.

Body composition FAQs

Q: To gain muscle, do I have to lift weights?

A: No. Weightlifting is one form of resistance exercise, but many other types of exercise that overload and put your muscles under 'stress' will also work your skeletal muscles. Exercises that use your own body weight as resistance can also build muscle, including circuit training, pilates and the use of stretch bands. Household items like cans or bottles can also be used as weights or dumbbells. However, over time as the body adapts to a resistance load, the level of resistance may have to increase to continue to see improvements. This is when heavier weights such as dumbbells can come in handy.

Q: Is the timing of protein intake important when doing resistance training? Does the 'post-exercise protein dose' matter?

A: There is some evidence that suggests having protein about 1 hour before or after exercise can have a very small beneficial effect. It can increase the 'thermic effect' of that protein (that is, the amount of energy it takes to actually digest food — see page 23), which can burn more kilojoules. However, this additional benefit to muscle gain is relatively small, so choose your meal timing based on what fits with your lifestyle. Ensuring you are simply eating adequate amounts of protein spread evenly across the day is the more important factor to focus on.

Q: Will resistance exercise training dramatically increase my muscle bulk if I am a woman?

A: Men and women experience similar proportional strength gains when training under the same resistance exercise program. However, in women, there appears to be less muscle mass gain compared to men. Simply put, women do not 'bulk up' like men. There is also no evidence that women need to train differently to men when undertaking resistance exercise.

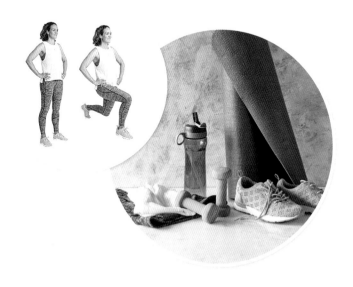

Achieving a healthy weight with protein

If you are trying to achieve a healthier weight, an energy-restricted, higher-protein diet can help you maximise your fat loss while minimising the loss of lean mass, particularly when undertaking a program of resistance exercise. Increasing your intake of dietary protein also offers additional benefits that can help you control your weight.

Protein helps manage appetite

The regulation of appetite is a complex system that involves a number of different hormones being released from the gut and other parts of the body, some of which are detailed below. These hormones have overlapping effects in a number of regions of the brain to modulate our drive to eat, feelings of fullness and satiety, along with other aspects of metabolism, such as blood glucose control. Some hormones increase our appetite and others suppress it.

Compared to meals higher in carbohydrate and fat, meals that are higher in protein have been shown to reduce feelings of hunger, boost fullness and satiation in the short term, and decrease subsequent food intake. This effect is linked to protein having specific effects on some of these appetite-regulating hormones.

Protein helps reduce food cravings

The body has a strong biological drive to seek protein. According to the 'protein leverage hypothesis' developed by Simpson and Raubenheimer, we are biologically primed to prioritise protein intake, and will keep consuming food until our essential amino acid needs are met.

Increases in the proportion of protein provided in meals have been shown to lower the desire to eat more carbohydrates and fats. Studies have also shown that after a high-protein breakfast, there is a more favourable suppression of nerve activation in the area of the brain that controls pleasure, cravings and the motivation to eat, compared to a high-carbohydrate breakfast. In other words, if we eat sufficient amounts of protein we are less likely to experience the drive to keep eating, which can cause us to over-consume.

However, to reap these subtle benefits, we must also be aware of, and appropriately respond to, our appetite cues. This can be challenging when we are faced with an abundant supply of highly palatable food, and when eating is such an ingrained part of our lifestyle. So it is important to listen to your body and stop eating when you feel full.

Hormone	Produced mainly by	Effect on appetite
Ghrelin	Stomach	Stimulatory
Leptin	Fat cells	Inhibitory
Cholecystokinin	Small intestine	Inhibitory
Peptide YY	Lower sections of the gastrointestinal tract	Inhibitory
Glucagon like peptide 1 and 2	Small intestine	Inhibitory

Protein helps boost metabolism

There are three main uses for energy in our body. The biggest proportion of our body's energy goes towards our **basal metabolic rate** — the energy our body uses even when it is at rest, to keep us alive.

The second (and most variable) component is the amount of energy used for physical activity.

The smallest component is the energy needed to digest, absorb and metabolise nutrients from our food and beverages. This is called the **thermic effect of food** (TEF). Approximately 10% of the kilojoules we consume are used for food digestion and the metabolism of absorbed nutrients.

The TEF for different food components varies. **Fats and carbohydrates** are very easy to metabolise, and so they have a lower thermic effect; approximately 5–15% of kilojoules consumed are used for fat and carbohydrate digestion. **Protein** requires more energy to digest and absorb, so it has a larger thermic effect; approximately 20–35% of kilojoules consumed are required to digest and metabolise protein.

There are some additional factors that can also help to increase the TEF, albeit in small ways. The thermic effect of food is higher:

* in the morning, compared with the evening
* when following a regular meal pattern
* in people participating in regular aerobic and resistance exercise.

Putting this information together, to maximise this natural thermic effect, there is some advantage to enjoying a reasonable-sized breakfast, having meals at regular times of the day, and ensuring that meals are relatively high in protein. This advantage relates to more kilojoules being used for food digestion and metabolism.

But remember, this is a relatively small effect. Consuming fewer kilojoules overall has a much bigger impact in creating an energy deficit to achieve weight loss.

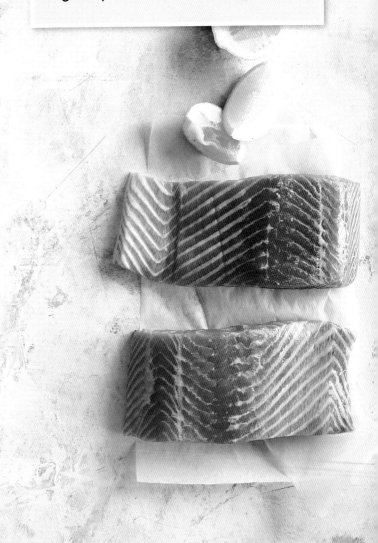

In summary, higher protein diets are advantageous for weight loss by helping control appetite and cravings, and contributing to an energy deficit. Pages 48–49 provide sample meal plans for higher-protein diets for weight loss.

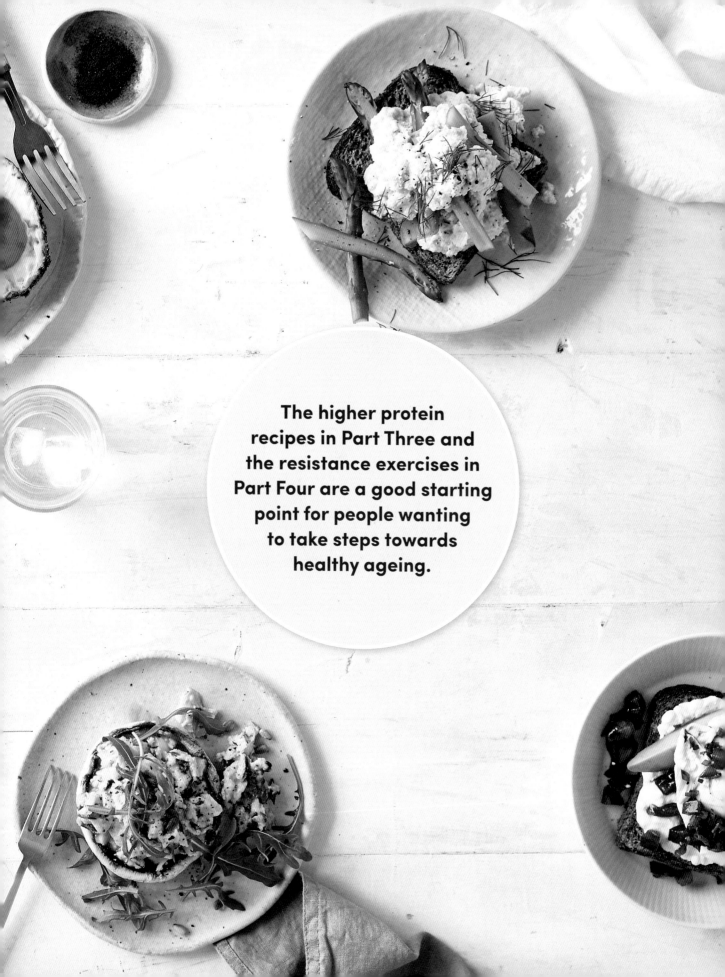

The higher protein recipes in Part Three and the resistance exercises in Part Four are a good starting point for people wanting to take steps towards healthy ageing.

Protein for healthy ageing

There are many changes that come with advancing age; hair and hearing loss and wrinkling skin are obvious ones. However, one that often goes unrecognised is the decline in skeletal muscle mass and strength.

It is unclear when it begins, but likely after the age of 40, our skeletal muscle mass decreases by 3–8% every decade. After the age of 60 it decreases by 10–15% per decade, or 1–1.5% every year. This rate of muscle decline can vary between individuals, but is exacerbated by a sedentary lifestyle, a low dietary protein intake, obesity and potentially genetics. At the same time as our muscle mass decreases, the fat content in our muscles increases, further contributing to poor muscle function, loss of strength and frailty.

This age-related loss of muscle mass, both in quantity and quality (i.e. strength and performance), is called **sarcopenia**. It reduces quality of life, decreases the ability to perform general daily activities, and increases the risk of falls and fractures, as well as premature death. Muscle mass loss occurs in all people as they age to varying extents, regardless of whether their body weight is high or low, and often goes unrecognised in people with a higher body weight.

Preserving muscle function as we age

The good news is that there are things we can all do to minimise the loss of muscle quantity and quality, no matter our age. **The combination of adequate dietary protein and regular resistance exercise can improve muscle mass and strength.**

It also appears that the *amount* and *type* of dietary protein also matters. As we age, our skeletal muscle seems to become less responsive to dietary protein — however, studies have shown that muscle-protein synthesis is stimulated after eating higher-quality proteins (such as dairy, eggs, meat, chicken and fish).

What's more, it's never too late — or too early! — to improve your eating and physical activity habits to protect your muscles. A recent review of 10 studies found that muscle mass increased in adults aged 60–80 years when they introduced resistance exercise and consumed extra protein from dairy foods.

EMERGING PROTEIN SCIENCE: Leucine may boost muscle protein synthesis

Recent studies have shown that one particular essential amino acid, leucine, may help to increase muscle protein synthesis and minimise muscle protein degradation. Studies have shown that leucine-rich proteins (such as whey from dairy) are more effective at building muscle than equivalent quantities of proteins that are lower in leucine.

To date, most studies have been performed in older adults, who are at increased risk of muscle loss and have a reduced response to the effects of dietary protein. Findings suggest that a leucine dose of around 2–3 grams per meal may enhance muscle protein synthesis; however, research is ongoing to see whether this also results in improved muscle strength and functionality. Because the effect of leucine appears to be more pronounced in older adults with a low muscle mass, scientists are continuing to investigate if leucine may play a beneficial role in healthy ageing.

Getting enough protein in plant-based diets

In Australia, the number of people choosing a total or partial vegetarian diet is growing. There are various reasons for this, including animal welfare issues, environmental concerns and a perception that these diets are better for our health.

Vegetarian diets exclude the consumption of all types of meat, meat products, fish and seafood. Dairy products, eggs and honey may or may not be included.

Lacto-ovo-vegetarian diets exclude meat, but include dairy products, eggs and honey, together with a wide variety of plant foods. Sub-categories are lacto-vegetarian, which excludes eggs, and ovo-vegetarian, which excludes dairy products.

Vegan diets exclude all meat, as well as dairy products, eggs, gelatin and honey, as these are sourced from animals.

In addition to vegetarian and vegan diets, an increasing number of people are choosing to eat meat and animal products less frequently (flexitarians), while some vegetarians choose to incorporate seafood (pescetarians).

Vegetarian diets and health

Vegetarian diets, like omnivorous diets (non-vegetarian diets that include a mixture of plant and animal-based foods), can be either healthy or unhealthy, depending on which foods are regularly consumed.

A vegetarian or vegan diet containing foods that are highly processed, low in fibre, and high in kilojoules, sugar, salt and unhealthy fats will not provide health benefits solely due to the absence of animal-derived products.

However, reviews of the studies on this topic tend to show that people who follow vegetarian diets long term have a lower risk of some cancers and some lifestyle-related diseases, such as heart disease.

While the health benefits of vegetarian diets are often assumed to be related to the avoidance of meat, these diets are also typically higher in other nutritious foods, particularly vegetables, nuts and seeds. People who follow vegetarian diets also generally have healthier lifestyles. So the long-term health benefits associated with vegetarian diets are likely to be due to a combination of dietary and lifestyle factors and not necessarily the avoidance of meat.

Well-planned vegetarian diets that include a wide variety of plant foods, adequate kilojoules and reliable sources of vitamin B12 (found in animal products such as meat, seafood, eggs and dairy, and in some fortified foods e.g. breakfast cereals) are able to meet most nutrient requirements — with three exceptions: vitamin D and long-chain omega-3 fats, plus the additional iron required during pregnancy. If not well-balanced, vegetarian diets can also be limited in protein, zinc and calcium.

Therefore, people who follow a vegetarian or vegan diet should consider:

* supplementing their diet with a reliable source of vitamin B12, such as vitamin-fortified foods or supplements, particularly people who choose a vegan diet
* regularly consuming good sources of calcium, iron and zinc, either as supplements, or fortified foods such as calcium-fortified soy milk, iron-fortified cereals and bread and fortified yeast spread
* regularly eating good plant sources of omega-3 fatty acids (such as walnuts, flax seeds, chia seeds and their oils), limiting linoleic acid intake (found in corn and sunflower oils), and taking an omega-3 supplement (EPA and DHA) to ensure good omega-3 status.

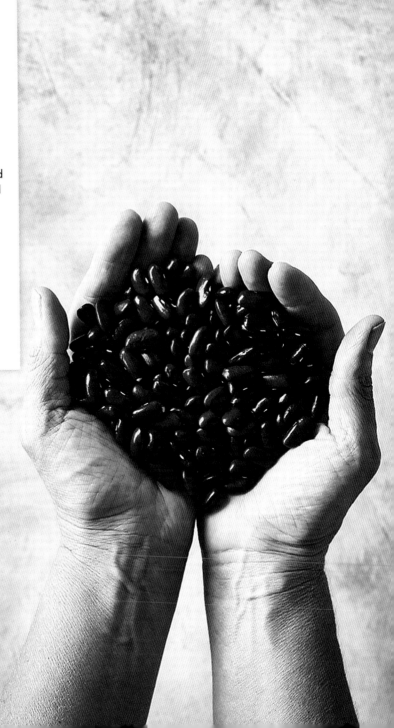

EMERGING PROTEIN SCIENCE:
The future of novel dietary proteins

Meeting the growing global population's needs for dietary protein and other nutrients into the future is predicted to be a challenge. Increasingly, alternative and novel dietary proteins are being put forward as possible solutions.

Farming insects that are fed on food waste is one option, although there are some production, consumer acceptance and regulatory hurdles to overcome.

Another option showing promise is to mimic animal proteins, such as beef. By using innovative food technologies that combine plant-based proteins and fibres with fermented compounds, food technologists have produced plant-based foods that have the look, taste, aroma and cooking properties of meat. More development is needed to enhance the nutritional profile of these alternate proteins, along with building consumer acceptance and demand.

Plant-based protein isolates from fava beans, peas, chia, hemp and quinoa could also be utilised more to address this challenge.

Plant-based proteins

As we saw on page 13, the quality of a dietary protein is determined by its amino acid content and digestibility. Most plant-based proteins (except soy) lack one or more essential amino acids and are generally lower in protein. Most also contain a significant amount of dietary fibre which, while an important nutrient, can reduce the body's ability to access, digest and utilise dietary protein. Plant-based proteins also often contain tannins, which interfere with protein digestion and amino acid absorption.

However, consuming a variety of plant foods can supply enough essential amino acids to ensure an adequate protein intake for vegetarians, especially if nuts, legumes and soy products are regularly consumed. In Australia, people who follow vegetarian and vegan diets generally meet or exceed current recommended protein intakes, when kilojoule intakes are adequate. However, plant-based proteins do not contain the same levels of iron, zinc, B12 and omega-3.

This book includes some higher protein recipes suitable for lacto-ovo vegetarians, along with many that can be easily adapted to suit.

Soy – a good source of plant protein

Soy-based products (such as soy milk, soy yoghurt and tofu) are some of the few plant-based protein sources that are similar in quality to animal proteins like eggs and cow's milk. Soy is considered higher quality because it is a complete protein (i.e. it contains all the essential amino acids), and soy-protein extracts are well digested and absorbed by our body. Some confusion exists over whether soy is healthy or not. This centres around isoflavones, which are natural plant chemicals found in soy. Isoflavones mimic some of the effects of oestrogen, although with a much weaker effect. However, current evidence from human studies does not show that soy foods consumed as part of a healthy diet cause any harm. In fact, there are a number of potential health benefits to regular soy consumption, including protection against heart disease and suggestive evidence of a reduced risk of certain cancers. Soy consumption is also consistent with the Australian Dietary Guidelines recommendation to eat a diet rich in plant foods.

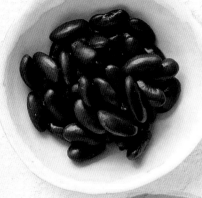

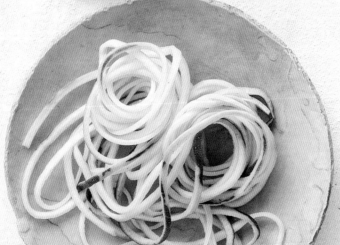

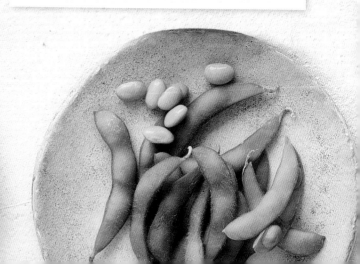

Diet, protein foods and the environment

Climate change is a pressing topic for scientists, the media and the general public. The global food system has a significant environmental impact, currently estimated to contribute 19–29% of global greenhouse gas emissions, and account for about 70% of global freshwater use. Despite these environmental costs, somewhere between 30–50% of all food produced is either not eaten or goes to waste. This loss occurs at each stage: from production, processing, distribution and retail, to us at home.

At CSIRO, we have looked into the greenhouse gas emissions attributed to the typical Australian diet. Discretionary foods (cakes, biscuits, chips and other foods and drinks that are high in sugar, saturated fats and salt, and low in nutrients) contribute almost one-third (29%) of the total greenhouse gas emissions in the average Australian diet, and contribute to excess energy intake. These foods provide very little nutritional value, so cutting back on the amount of these we consume has the double benefit of helping to lower our environmental impact and improve our diet quality.

In our analysis, fresh meats (such as red meat, poultry and fish) also contribute approximately one-third (32%) of greenhouse gas emissions that are attributed to diet, but they provide many beneficial nutrients, including high-quality protein, leucine, iron, B12 and zinc. Given the importance of consuming a nutrient-dense diet, we can make a difference to the environment by not wasting food, and not consuming more than we need.

Following a partial or completely vegetarian diet is a strategy that some people choose to help reduce their carbon footprint. While this choice is not for everyone, we can all help reduce the environmental impact of the food system by:

* consuming fewer discretionary ('junk') foods and beverages
* minimising food waste
* not eating more food than our body needs.

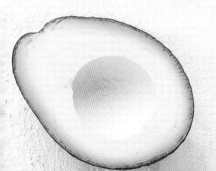
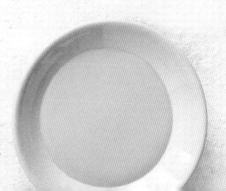
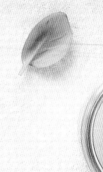

Spreading out your protein intake to boost the benefits

There is evidence demonstrating the benefits of a higher protein intake for improving body composition, supporting weight loss and promoting healthy ageing. In addition, in the past few years some exciting new evidence has emerged from leading research laboratories around the world, suggesting that spreading your intake of dietary protein across the day adds extra benefit.

Typically, Australians eat most of their dietary protein towards the end of the day at the evening meal, and little at the beginning of the day. Some studies have shown that distributing protein intake more evenly across the day — with a focus on increasing the amount of protein consumed at breakfast — may further optimise the benefits and health effects of a higher-protein diet.

The graphs below highlight the difference between **the current daily distribution of dietary protein** in the average Australian diet (based on the latest national nutrition survey), and **a more evenly distributed protein intake** supported by recent scientific evidence.

Appetite regulation to assist body weight control

Single-meal studies have consistently shown that, compared to eating a meal rich in either carbohydrate or fat, a high-protein meal more effectively increases feelings of fullness in the short-term, reduces hunger and decreases the amount of food you eat at the next meal. Many studies have tested this effect at breakfast.

Based on this evidence, increasing the amount of protein consumed at each meal across the day could help to prolong these appetite-suppressing effects, and in turn this can help to reduce our overall food and energy intake each day.

Muscle protein synthesis for improved muscle mass and function

Muscle protein synthesis is the biological process that occurs to build and maintain muscle in the body. Several short-term studies have compared the effects of different distributions of a set amount of total daily dietary protein — either in a skewed distribution (with most of the protein consumed in the evening meal and a little at lunch and breakfast), or evenly spread across the day.

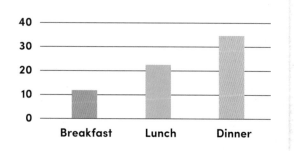

Current 'skewed' intake of protein (g) per day

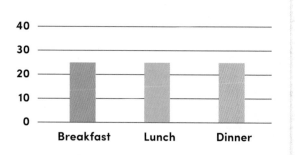

Evenly distributed intake of protein (g) per day

The more even distribution is associated with higher total muscle protein synthesis (building new muscle). If too little protein is consumed at one time, muscle protein synthesis is not sufficiently stimulated. And if excess dietary protein is consumed above the amount used for muscle synthesis, it is of limited benefit because it cannot be stored and used at a later time to build muscle. Studies suggest that consuming about 25 grams of high quality dietary protein per meal is a good guide.

Based on this emerging information, leading scientists in this field suggest that more evenly distributing protein across your meals throughout the day could promote greater muscle mass and strength gains over the longer term.

Further research is being undertaken to confirm and understand how much additional benefit can be gained from consuming protein with an even distribution pattern. Nevertheless, this strategy may help optimise the benefits that can be achieved from a higher-protein diet, especially when combined with resistance exercise training.

How much dietary protein do Australians consume?

The Australian National Nutrition and Health Survey conducted in 2012 shows that the average protein intake per day for adults is above the current Australian RDI and closer to the amounts supported by recent research. Good news!

The downside is that this higher protein intake is within diets that are also high in energy from discretionary foods. In fact, almost one-third of our energy comes from high-energy, nutrient-poor foods and drinks, high in refined sugars, salt and saturated fats — or alcohol. And just 24% of women and 15% of men meet the target of two serves of fruit and five serves of vegetables a day.

In other words, while most Australian adults may be consuming adequate amounts of dietary protein, they are also consuming too much food (i.e. energy) overall. This, along with a sedentary lifestyle, is contributing to our nation's high — and increasing — rates of obesity in adults. We also see that the average daily protein intake is lower in both females and males aged over 70 years, even though the Australian Dietary Guidelines and latest scientific evidence recommend high protein for this age group.

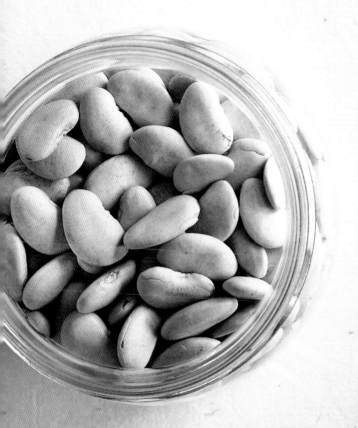

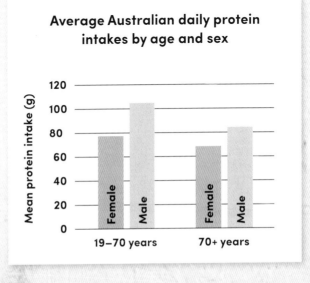

Average Australian daily protein intakes by age and sex

When do Australians eat protein?

These national nutrition survey results also show that Australian adults eat almost half of their total daily protein at the evening meal — on average, 38 grams of protein. In contrast, the average amount of protein consumed at breakfast is less than 15 grams. Interestingly, food eaten outside of the three main meals contributes almost one-fifth of our protein intake — which is more than breakfast, and highlights just how much Australians snack throughout the day.

Average dietary protein intake by meal occasion and age group

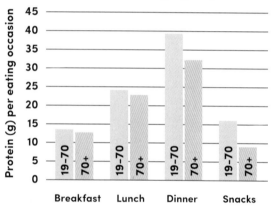

Protein sources in the Australian diet

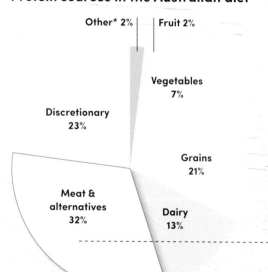

Where does our dietary protein come from?

The survey shows that we get our protein from a range of foods (see pie charts below). Some of these foods are what you might expect to be key sources of protein in our diet, such as meat and dairy foods. However, the 'discretionary' food group is the second biggest contributor to protein intake, at 23%. This group consists of foods such as processed meats, pizza, savoury and sweet pastries, cakes and biscuits. Processed meats, such as sausages, commercial burgers, ham and other cured meats, are considered discretionary foods because of their high saturated fat and salt content. Despite being relatively low in protein, these discretionary foods are a big contributor to our total protein intake because they are eaten frequently and in large quantities. This is partly why Australians are consuming so much extra energy. If we ate more protein from core food groups and less discretionary foods, it would be easier to meet our protein needs without having to consume those 'empty' kilojoules that can contribute to weight gain.

In the 'meat and alternatives' group, the survey shows that red meat is the most consumed protein, while fish and vegetarian alternatives make relatively small contributions to dietary protein intake. Current recommendations are to consume no more than 455 grams (cooked weight) of lean red meat per week. So whilst red meat is a popular choice and an important source of nutrients, it is better to consume a variety of other dietary proteins as well, including white meat, fish, seafood, eggs, dairy and plant-based proteins.

Sources of meat and alternatives

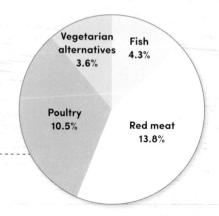

* 'Other' includes a range of miscellaneous foods like fats, oils, herbs and spices

In summary, **Australians are consuming too many kilojoules** (energy), particularly from discretionary foods, and from food and drinks consumed outside of mealtimes.

The recipes in this book will help you to meet your protein requirements, using a variety of protein sources and primarily including foods from nutrient-rich core food groups.

They will also show how you can distribute your protein intake more evenly throughout the day, and increase your protein intake at breakfast.

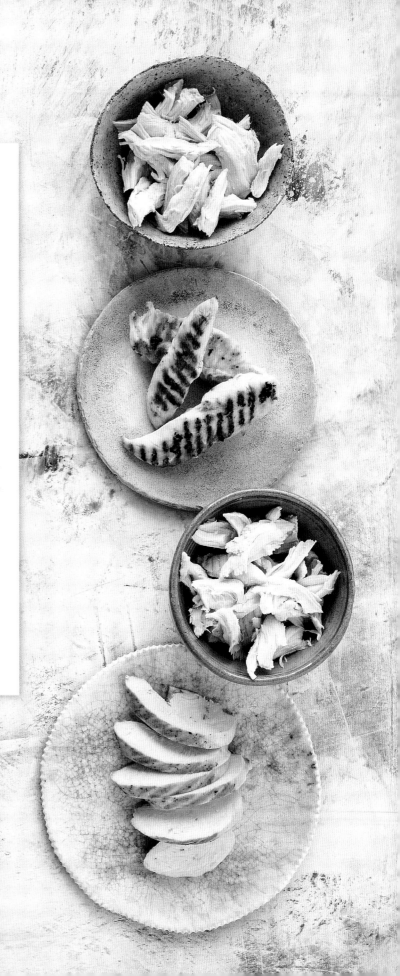

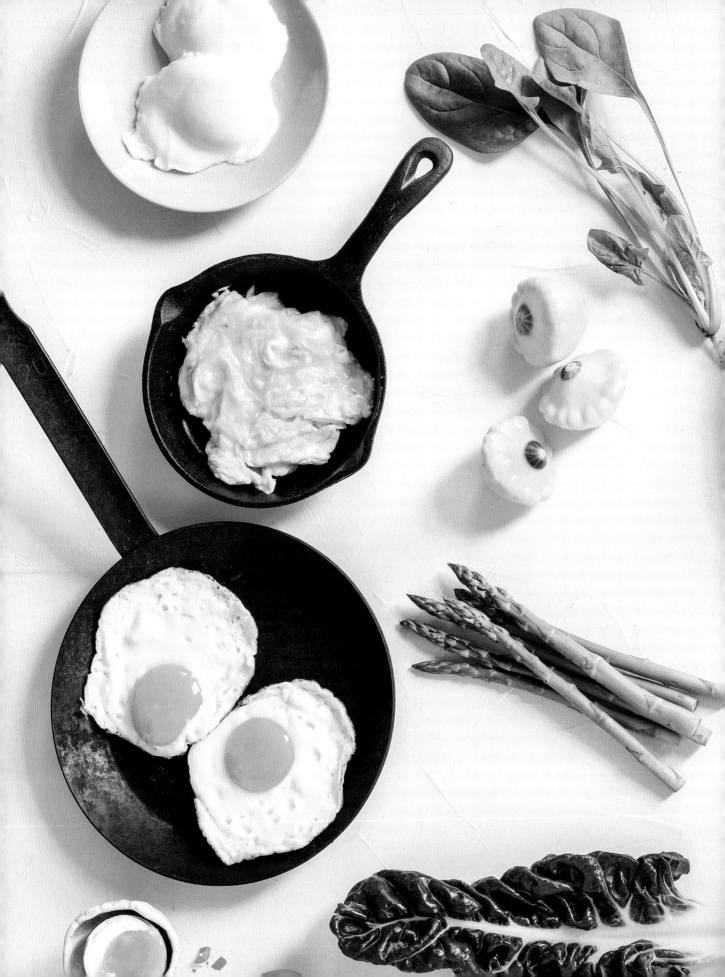

In Part One, we outlined the scientific principles supporting a higher dietary protein intake, as well as the emerging evidence about the benefits of evenly distributing dietary protein across the days' main meals.

The sample meal plans provided in **Part Two** illustrate how this information can be incorporated into an overall eating plan.

Part Three provides a collection of breakfast, lunch and dinner recipes (see page 56), which can be used to achieve a healthy, higher-protein eating pattern with protein spread evenly throughout the day.

To get more out of this higher dietary protein approach, a resistance exercise plan is also included in **Part Four** (page 242). This simple, practical program can be followed by anyone wishing to improve their body composition, physical strength and wellbeing – whether you are trying to lose weight, build muscle mass, maintain muscle mass, age healthily or any combination of the above.

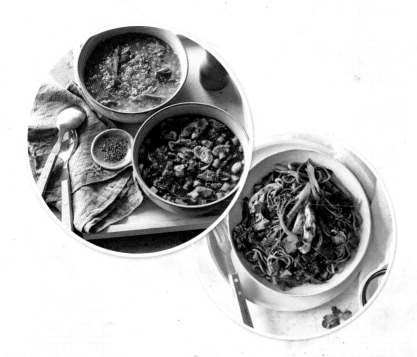

Remember to consult your doctor before beginning a diet and exercise program.

PART TWO

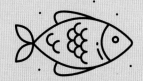

Realising the Power of Protein

How to use this book to boost your protein intake with an even daily distribution

As we have described in Part One, a higher dietary-protein intake that is more evenly spread across breakfast, lunch and dinner, combined with regular resistance exercises, helps to maintain muscle mass, improve body composition and support healthy ageing, and can also aid weight loss.

The key to achieving a balanced, nutritious diet is to select a variety of foods from each of the core food groups. These foods should make up the greatest part of what we eat, and are key features of the recipes and sample meal plans in this book.

The tables on the following pages summarise the key nutrition information for the core food groups. This information includes the average protein content of these foods so that comparisons can be made between food groups.

It is also important to limit discretionary foods, as they are high in added sugar, salt, saturated fats or alcohol, and low in beneficial nutrients. Processed meats – such as ham, bacon, prosciutto and other cured meats, sausages, hot dogs and commercial burgers – are high in unhealthy fats and salt and, as such, are considered discretionary foods, even though they provide some protein.

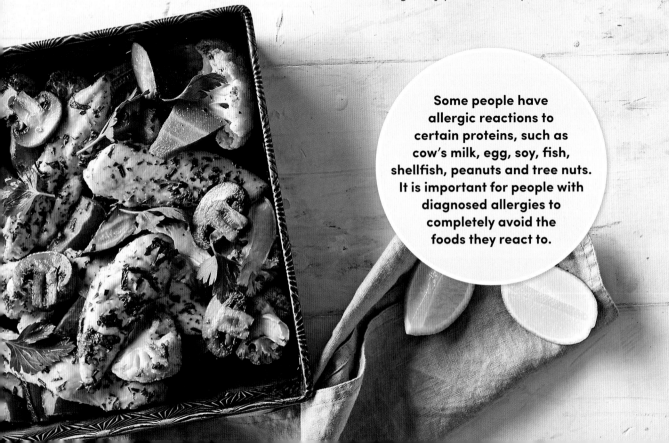

Some people have allergic reactions to certain proteins, such as cow's milk, egg, soy, fish, shellfish, peanuts and tree nuts. It is important for people with diagnosed allergies to completely avoid the foods they react to.

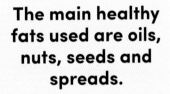

The main sources of protein in these recipes are:

* **Meat and alternatives** — lean red meat, fish, chicken, eggs, legumes and other vegetarian options

* **Dairy and soy** or other high-protein dairy substitutes (choose low-fat milks and yoghurts)

Low-kilojoule vegetables are an important feature of most recipes.

They provide fibre, vitamins and minerals, along with flavour, colour, texture and bulk.

The main healthy fats used are oils, nuts, seeds and spreads.

These are energy-dense, so should be used in small quantities.

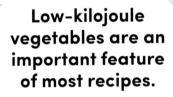

The main carbohydrate and fibre sources provide smaller amounts of protein:

* **Low-GI and wholegrain**, or fibre-enriched, bread/cereal foods

* **Fruit**

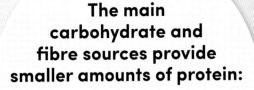

Core food groups and serving sizes

This table summarises the core food groups and recommended serving sizes used as the basis for the recipes and sample meal plans in this book. It also shows the average protein and energy content of the foods, so you can make comparisons between items and between core food groups. These food groups are similar to those set by the Australian Guide to Healthy Eating (**eatforhealth.gov.au**). The only differences here are that nuts come under the OILS category because they are lower in protein, and starchy vegetables are in the GRAINS category because they are higher in carbohydrate and energy.

CORE FOOD GROUPS	AVERAGE PROTEIN (G)	AVERAGE ENERGY (KJ)	KEY NUTRIENTS	RECOMMENDATIONS
GRAINS **Mainly low-GI, wholegrain choices:**			Slow-release, low-GI carbohydrates, folate, fibre and B-group vitamins.	Choose wholegrain or wholemeal options that are higher in fibre, more nutritious and can have a lower GI, which will help to keep you feeling fuller for longer. Note: 150 g starchy vegetables such as potato/sweet potato can be swapped for a grain serve.
* 1 slice bread (40 g) or ½ bread roll	4.5	417		
* 1 slice fruit loaf	2.8	391		
* 1 crumpet (60 g)	3.2	523		
* 3 high-fibre crispbreads (e.g. Ryvita)	3.7	550		
* ½ cup (75–120 g) cooked rice, pasta, noodles, barley, buckwheat, semolina, polenta, burghul or quinoa	2.6–5.4	395–640		
* ⅔ cup (30 g) high-fibre breakfast cereal (e.g. Sultana Bran, Fibre Plus)	3.2	395		
* ½ cup (120 g) cooked porridge (⅓ cup oats cooked in water)	3.1	517		
* ¼ cup (30 g) muesli	3.4	513		

Glycaemic index (GI) is a scale comparing foods based on their likelihood of raising blood glucose. Foods are given a GI of 1 to 100 based on the total rise of blood glucose after consumption, compared to pure glucose, which is set at 100.

CORE FOOD GROUPS	AVERAGE PROTEIN (G)	AVERAGE ENERGY (KJ)	KEY NUTRIENTS	RECOMMENDATIONS
DAIRY & alternatives				
✷ 1 cup (250 ml) low-fat milk	9.4	497	Protein, calcium, vitamin B12, iodine, zinc and vitamin B2. Dairy (except most cheeses) also provides carbohydrates. Some dairy alternatives are fortified with vitamin B12 and calcium.	Choose low-fat milk and yoghurt, to limit saturated fat and energy (kilojoules). *Rice milk and almond milk are not equivalent in protein content to dairy milk. We suggest adding 1 tablespoon (approx 10 g) of vegetable-based protein powder per 1 cup (250 ml) of rice/almond beverages.
✷ 1 cup (250 ml) unsweetened soy milk with at least 100 mg added calcium per 100 ml*	7.7	404		
✷ ½ cup (120 ml) evaporated skim milk	10.5	428		
✷ 200 g tub of low-fat or diet yoghurt	15.0	752		
✷ 200 g tub of low-fat custard or dairy dessert	7.6	692		
✷ 2 x 20 g slices or a 40 g serve of hard cheese, such as cheddar	9.8	665		
✷ ½ cup (120 g) ricotta cheese or cottage cheese	12.2	635		
MEAT & alternatives				
✷ 100 g chicken (raw weight); or 80 g cooked chicken	22.3	438	Protein • Meats are higher in zinc and iron • Animal proteins provide vitamin B12 • Legumes contain fibre • Oily fish provide healthy omega-3 fats	Choose lean cuts of meat, and trim off visible fat and remove skin, to reduce the saturated fat and energy (kilojoule) content. Avoid processed meats, e.g. bacon, which are high in salt. Choose tinned beans or legumes with no added salt. Aim for up to 455 g of red meat per week. Aim for two fish or seafood meals per week.
✷ 100 g turkey (raw weight); or 80 g cooked turkey	21.6	490		
✷ 100 g pork (raw weight); or 80 g cooked pork	22.8	502		
✷ 100 g beef (raw weight); or 80 g cooked beef	27.8	587		
✷ 100 g lamb (raw weight); or 80 g cooked lamb	21.2	566		
✷ 100 g tinned or fresh fish or seafood	22.0	440		
✷ 2 large eggs	12.6	533		
✷ 1 cup (150 g) cooked or tinned legumes	9.6	639		
✷ 170 g firm tofu	20.4	853		
✷ 100 g Quorn™	20.0	849		

CORE FOOD GROUPS	AVERAGE PROTEIN (G)	AVERAGE ENERGY (KJ)	KEY NUTRIENTS	RECOMMENDATIONS
FRUIT				
* 1 medium apple, banana, orange or pear	<1	350	Carbohydrates (as natural fruit sugars), vitamin C, folate, potassium and dietary fibre.	Choose whole fruit in preference to dried fruit or juice. Whole fruit contains more fibre than juice, and has a higher water content making it more filling than dried fruit. Juice and dried fruit can also increase the risk of dental decay because of the concentrated sugar and acidity of juice.
* 2 small apricots, kiwi fruit or plums	<1	350		
* 1 cup diced or tinned fruit (no added sugar)	<1	350		
* 150 ml unsweetened fruit juice (occasionally)	<1	350		
* 30 g dried fruit (e.g. 4 dried apricot halves or 1½ tablespoons sultanas)	<1	350		
VEGETABLES				
* ½ cup cooked vegetables*	1–6	100–150	Fibre, folate, vitamins A, B6 and C, magnesium, beta-carotene and antioxidants.	Choose a variety of colours and a mixture of salad and cooked vegetables. Fresh, frozen and tinned vegetables can be used. If using tinned vegetables, look for varieties with no added salt.
* 1 cup green leafy or raw salad vegetables* * Choosing from the free list on page 52	<1	100		
OILS, nuts & spreads				
* 1 teaspoon liquid oil (canola, olive, sunflower)	0	170	Vitamins A, E and K, antioxidants and omega-3 and omega-6 fats.	Choose from any unsaturated fats and oils including olive oil, canola oil, sunflower oil, avocadoes, nuts and seeds.
* 1 teaspoon soft margarine (trans-fat free)	0	100		
* 2 teaspoons light (reduced-fat) margarine	0	100		
* 1 tablespoon curry paste in oil	<1	200		
* 1 tablespoon (20 g) avocado	<1	170		
* 7 g nuts or seeds	1.5	170		
Note: A small amount of spray oil is a 'free' item.				

One way to use this book is to simply start incorporating some of the recipes in Part Three into your cooking repertoire for breakfast, lunch and dinner.

Each recipe provides at least 25 grams of protein, which sets a good foundation for meeting the protein requirements of most healthy adults, and will help you to achieve a more evenly distributed protein intake throughout the day. In addition, the recipes are based on the core food groups, so they are high in fibre and vegetables and low in refined carbohydrates, sugars and salt, and contain healthy fats and some wholegrain carbohydrates, making them nutrient-dense and suitable for long-term good health.

* **Breakfast**: The typical Australian breakfast is usually based on carbohydrate-containing foods, such as toast and cereal, and is therefore often low in dietary protein. The breakfast recipes in this book will boost the dietary protein content of this meal by including ingredients such as low-fat milk, yoghurt, cheese, eggs and legumes. The recipes still include wholegrain cereals or bread, but as an accompaniment rather than being central to the dish.
* **Lunch**: The lunch recipes flip the usual proportions of carbohydrate to protein foods and reduce the proportion of carbohydrate-based foods in favour of larger amounts of protein-rich foods. They also contain a generous helping of salad and/or vegetables, which add flavour, texture, variety, fibre and lots of nutrients to help you power through the day.
* **Dinner**: Low-starch vegetables, along with a variety of protein-rich foods, are the key features here. Small amounts of wholegrains and healthy fats are also used in these recipes. Wholegrains and higher starch vegetables can be added as an accompaniment, depending on your energy needs.

The recipes use a variety of animal- and plant-based proteins to suit different eating styles and preferences. Some of the meat-based recipes can also be modified using a vegetarian or vegan alternative, such as tofu, tempeh and vegetarian mince or nuggets. Vegetarian proteins require different cooking times and sometimes different cooking methods to meat, so adjust accordingly. Most importantly of all, the meals are practical, easy to make and delicious.

Sample meal plans

If you are looking for a more structured approach, the other way this book can be used is to follow the sample meal plans.

Throughout our years of research at CSIRO, we have learned a lot about the many elements that contribute to successful, long-term improvements in dietary habits. We know that adjusting your food and energy intake – while at the same time achieving a nutritionally balanced and satisfying diet – is difficult to do on your own. Our experience has shown that clear, meal-based plans are a critical element to enable people to form healthier eating habits.

For this reason we have included some higher-protein meal plans that help you to achieve a more even distribution of your dietary protein across the day (25 grams protein at each meal), whilst also ensuring a balance of core food groups.

> **Understanding the beneficial effects of eating breakfast continues to remain an active area of scientific research. However, current evidence suggests a breakfast containing higher amounts of protein may have beneficial effects on weight management, body composition and healthy ageing.**

These meal plans indicate the number of serves, or 'units', of core foods allocated to breakfast, lunch and dinner meals (shown in the left-hand columns of the tables on pages 46–49), along with some allowance for snacks. The units are distributed in such a way to ensure that each main meal provides at least 25 grams of protein, and the recipes in this book match these meal allowances, making it easy to put the meal plan into practice.

The example foods shown in the right-hand column of the sample meal plans show how the units can be used without following a recipe from this book – because, let's face it, we don't always eat home-cooked meals. You can also use the unit allowance for each meal and select other options from the core food groups table (pages 40–42).

Remember, these meal plans are a guide. You may find that you need more or less food, depending on your body size and activity level. However, most people find it helpful to have a basic structure like this to help them form a healthy eating routine that can be followed long-term. For a more personalised approach, we recommend you consult an accredited practising dietitian, or consider the online CSIRO Total Wellbeing Diet which provides a simple, flexible 12-week Protein Balance weight loss program (totalwellbeingdiet.com).

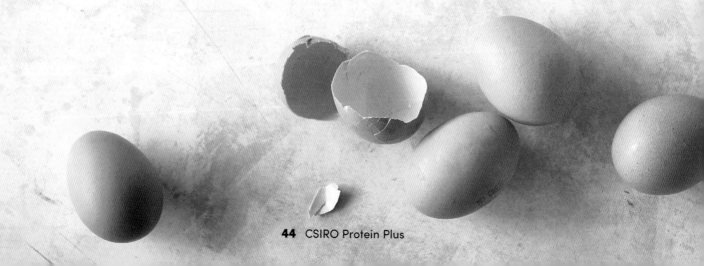

These meal plans offer two options to give some variety and suit different eating styles.

Sample Meal Plan A includes breakfasts that require less preparation, featuring smoothies or a more traditional 'toast or cereal' option. Lunch includes meat and alternatives. When following this meal plan, you will need to choose both Breakfast *and* Lunch recipes marked with an A.

Sample Meal Plan B features eggs or other protein foods at breakfast. Lunch includes dairy protein. When following this meal plan, you will need to choose both Breakfast *and* Lunch recipes marked with a B.

You can elect to follow either Plan A or B on different days of the week, as long as you stick with one plan for the whole day. For example, you might choose **Meal Plan A** for weekdays and **Meal Plan B** for weekends. Or you might simply prefer to always follow one particular meal plan. Don't worry if you occasionally mix A and B meals on the same day: you will still be achieving 25 grams of protein per meal and will only be consuming a few more or a few less kilojoules that day. Both meal plans have the same structure for the evening meal, so you can choose any dinner recipe, regardless of whether you are following Plan A or B!

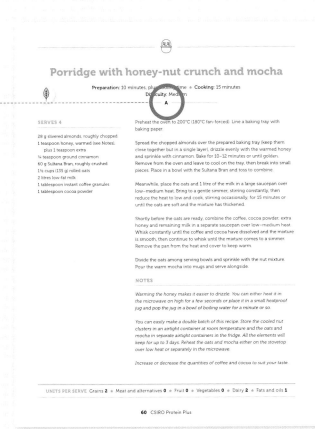

Porridge with honey-nut crunch and mocha

Preparation: 10 minutes, plus cooling time ● Cooking: 15 minutes
Difficulty: Medium

A

SERVES 4

28 g slivered almonds, roughly chopped
1 teaspoon honey, warmed (see Notes), plus 1 teaspoon extra
¼ teaspoon ground cinnamon
60 g Sultana Bran, roughly crushed
1½ cups (135 g) rolled oats
2 litres low-fat milk
1 tablespoon instant coffee granules
1 tablespoon cocoa powder

Preheat the oven to 200°C (180°C fan-forced). Line a baking tray with baking paper.

Spread the chopped almonds over the prepared baking tray (keep them close together but in a single layer), drizzle evenly with the warmed honey and sprinkle with cinnamon. Bake for 10–12 minutes or until golden. Remove from the oven and leave to cool on the tray, then break into small pieces. Place in a bowl with the Sultana Bran and toss to combine.

Meanwhile, place the oats and 1 litre of the milk in a large saucepan over low–medium heat. Bring to a gentle simmer, stirring constantly, then reduce the heat to low and cook, stirring occasionally, for 15 minutes or until the oats are soft and the mixture has thickened.

Shortly before the oats are ready, combine the coffee, cocoa powder, extra honey and remaining milk in a separate saucepan over low–medium heat. Whisk constantly until the coffee and cocoa have dissolved and the mixture is smooth, then continue to whisk until the mixture comes to a simmer. Remove the pan from the heat and cover to keep warm.

Divide the oats among serving bowls and sprinkle with the nut mixture. Pour the warm mocha into mugs and serve alongside.

NOTES

Warming the honey makes it easier to drizzle. You can either heat it in the microwave on high for a few seconds or place it in a small heatproof jug and pop the jug in a bowl of boiling water for a minute or so.

You can easily make a double batch of this recipe. Store the cooled nut clusters in an airtight container at room temperature and the oats and mocha in separate airtight containers in the fridge. All the elements will keep for up to 3 days. Reheat the oats and mocha either on the stovetop over low heat or separately in the microwave.

Increase or decrease the quantities of coffee and cocoa to suit your taste.

UNITS PER SERVE Grains **2** ● Meat and alternatives **0** ● Fruit **0** ● Vegetables **0** ● Dairy **2** ● Fats and oils **1**

60 CSIRO Protein Plus

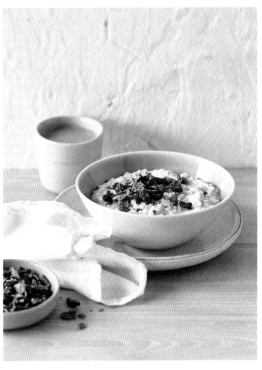

Breakfast **61**

Dietary protein for healthy eating

This table shows how you can structure meals and snacks to provide **8000 kJ** per day.
This moderate energy level is a starting point for a healthy eating plan for weight maintenance.
If you are very physically active or a bigger person, this is unlikely to be enough food for you.
For a more personalised approach, we recommend you consult an accredited practising dietitian.

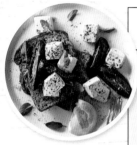

FOOD GROUP UNITS PER MEAL

SAMPLE MEAL PLAN A

BREAKFAST 2 Dairy 2 Grains 1 Oil	* 60 g high-fibre breakfast cereal served with 150 ml low-fat milk * 200 g low-fat yoghurt topped with 7 g slivered almonds * 100 ml low-fat milk (in coffee or tea)
LUNCH 1 Grain 1 Meat 2 Vege 1 Oil	* 1 slice wholegrain bread (40 g) * 2 cups garden salad dressed with vinegar and 1 teaspoon olive oil * 100 g chicken*
DINNER 1.5 Meat 3 Vege 2 Grains 1 Oil	* 150 g fish*, grilled, served with mixed vegetables stir-fried with ginger, Asian herbs * 1 cup cooked brown rice * 1 teaspoon oil, soy sauce To add grains to the dinner recipes in this book, refer to the core foods table on page 40 for serving sizes.
SNACKS 1 Dairy 3 Fruit 3 Oil	* 150 g fresh fruit salad * Apple with 1 tablespoon peanut butter * Banana smoothie made with 1 banana and 1 cup (250 ml) low-fat milk

TOTAL UNITS PER DAY		
	MEAT	2.5
	GRAINS	5
	DAIRY	3
	FRUIT	3
	VEGETABLES	5+
	OILS	6
	0–3 Indulgence foods per week (see page 50)	

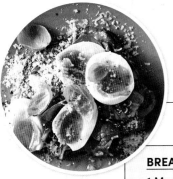
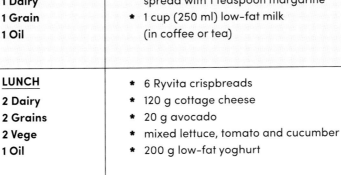

SAMPLE MEAL PLAN B

FOOD GROUP UNITS PER MEAL

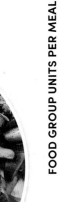

BREAKFAST

1 Meat
1 Dairy
1 Grain
1 Oil

* 2 large eggs
* 1 slice wholegrain bread (40 g), spread with 1 teaspoon margarine
* 1 cup (250 ml) low-fat milk (in coffee or tea)

LUNCH

2 Dairy
2 Grains
2 Vege
1 Oil

* 6 Ryvita crispbreads
* 120 g cottage cheese
* 20 g avocado
* mixed lettuce, tomato and cucumber
* 200 g low-fat yoghurt

DINNER

1.5 Meat
3 Vege
2 Grains
1 Oil

* 150 g beef*, barbecued
* coleslaw salad
* 1 cup cooked wholewheat couscous
* 1 teaspoon low-fat coleslaw dressing

To add grains to the dinner recipes in this book, refer to the core foods table on page 40 for serving sizes.

SNACKS

1 Dairy
3 Fruit
3 Oil

* 150 g fresh fruit salad
* Apple with 1 tablespoon peanut butter
* Banana smoothie made with 1 banana and 1 cup (250 ml) low-fat milk

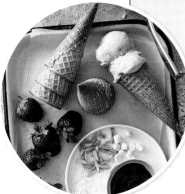

TOTAL UNITS PER DAY

MEAT	2.5
GRAINS	5
DAIRY	4
FRUIT	3
VEGETABLES	5+
OILS	6

0–3 Indulgence foods per week (see page 50)

Note: More information about the core food groups and serving sizes can be found on pages 40–42.

* This is the raw weight before cooking. It will weigh approximately 20% less after cooking.

Dietary protein for weight loss

This table shows how you can structure meals and snacks to provide **6000 kJ** per day. This low energy intake is a starting point for a diet aimed at achieving weight loss. If you are very physically active or a bigger person, this is unlikely to be enough food for you, even for weight loss. For a more personalised approach, we recommend you consult an accredited practising dietitian. The online CSIRO Total Wellbeing Diet also provides a simple, flexible 12-week Protein Balance weight-loss program (totalwellbeingdiet.com).

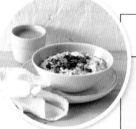

SAMPLE MEAL PLAN A

FOOD GROUP UNITS PER MEAL

BREAKFAST 2 Dairy 2 Grains 1 Oil	* 60 g high-fibre breakfast cereal served with 150 ml low-fat milk * 200 g low-fat yoghurt topped with 7 g slivered almonds * 100 ml low-fat milk (in coffee or tea)
LUNCH 1 Grain 1 Meat 2 Vege 1 Oil	* 1 slice wholegrain bread (40 g) * 2 cups garden salad dressed with vinegar and 1 teaspoon olive oil * 100 g chicken*
DINNER 1.5 Meat 3 Vege 1 Oil	* 150 g fish*, grilled * mixed vegetables stir-fried with ginger and Asian herbs * 1 teaspoon oil and soy sauce
SNACKS 1 Dairy 2 Fruit	* 1 cup (250 ml) low-fat milk (in coffee or tea) * 2 serves fruit * any free foods

TOTAL UNITS PER DAY		
	MEAT	2.5
	GRAINS	3
	DAIRY	3
	FRUIT	2
	VEGETABLES	5+
	OILS	3
	0–3 Indulgence foods per week (see page 50)	

And for some inspiring weight-loss tips, see page 53 for stories shared by our volunteers who have successfully achieved and maintained their weight-loss goals on a range of CSIRO higher-protein diets.

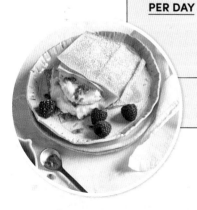

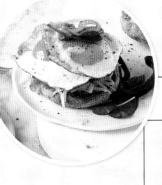

SAMPLE MEAL PLAN B

FOOD GROUP UNITS PER MEAL

BREAKFAST
1 Meat
1 Dairy
1 Grain
1 Oil

* 2 large eggs
* 1 slice wholegrain bread (40 g), spread with 1 teaspoon margarine
* 1 cup (250 ml) low-fat milk (in coffee or tea)

LUNCH
2 Dairy
2 Grains
2 Vege
1 Oil

* 6 Ryvita crispbreads
* 120 g cottage cheese
* 20 g avocado
* mixed lettuce, tomato and cucumber
* 200 g low-fat yoghurt

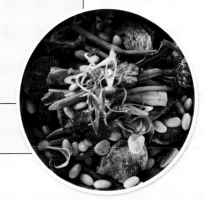

DINNER
1.5 Meat
3 Vege
1 Oil

* 150 g beef*, barbecued
* 3 cups garden salad, dressed with 1 teaspoon olive oil and vinegar

SNACKS
1 Dairy
2 Fruit

* 1 cup (250 ml) low-fat milk (in coffee or tea)
* 2 serves fruit
* any free foods

TOTAL UNITS PER DAY

MEAT	2.5
GRAINS	3
DAIRY	4
FRUIT	2
VEGETABLES	5+
OILS	3

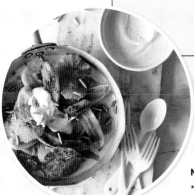

0–3 Indulgence foods per week (see page 50)

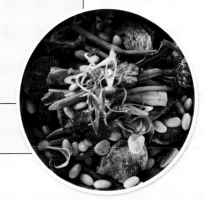

Note: More information about the core food groups and serving sizes can be found on pages 40–42.

* This is the raw weight before cooking. It will weigh approximately 20% less after cooking.

Between-meal snacks

For the average Australian adult, just over a quarter of our energy is consumed outside of main meals. Most of these snacks are discretionary foods and drinks – options that are low in nutritional quality and high in salt, added sugar, saturated fats and alcohol.

It is useful to consider that any between-meal snacks should be balanced with our energy needs. Snacks should be just that – a small amount of food, and therefore portion-controlled. Aim for no more than 400–600 kJ per snack. Snacks are an opportunity to boost our intake of foods that we tend to under-consume at main meals, such as fruit, vegetables and dairy, all of which adults struggle to eat enough of.

The sample meal plans in this book make an allowance for snacks, and it is up to individual preference as to when these are consumed. If you prefer not to eat in between meals, these foods can be added to your main meal allowance.

For people who eat between-meal snacks, you might consider our higher protein snack recipes (see pages 136–139). These portion-controlled snacks provide good sources of dietary protein and other beneficial nutrients, and can replace some of the commonly favoured discretionary snack choices.

Healthy indulgences

In this eating plan, up to three indulgence units are allowed per week. These can be spread across the week, or eaten all in one day or at one meal. One unit is any food or beverage of between approximately 400–600 kJ. You can choose to:

* use this allowance to enjoy some additional core foods, for example extra nuts, cheese, fruit or bread. This can be useful when dining out or eating with friends.
* try some of the Healthy Indulgence recipes on pages 222–241. These recipes contain mostly healthy ingredients, along with some indulgent additions, to create a nutritious and delicious finish to a meal. They are great for dinner parties or celebrations and can be used either as part of your weekly indulgences, or as extras for people not wanting to lose weight.

> **The recipes in the Healthy Indulgences chapter (page 222) can be enjoyed on the weight-loss plan (up to three indulgence units per week). The fruit units in these recipes also count towards your daily allowance.**

SNACK SWAPS	
Feel like?	**Go for:**
A cake or biscuit	Jaffa protein ball (page 139)
Potato chips	Roasted chickpeas (page 138)
Ice cream	Frozen yoghurt pops (page 139)
Chocolate mousse	Chia puddings with maple strawberries (page 139)
Muesli bar	Nut butter boat (page 136)
Cheese and biscuit	Herbed egg on crispbread (page 137)

Tips for healthy eating with your family

The way food is regarded within a family has a powerful influence on establishing healthy eating habits for our children and grandchildren. Here are some simple strategies that may help support healthy eating in your family.

* Try involving your children and family in planning the week's meals, creating shopping lists, then using the list in the supermarket or online. Share some of the choices with them, but limit the scope to answers you will be happy with. For example, 'Would you like stir-fry or a roast for dinner?' is preferable to 'What would you like for dinner?'
* Encourage your children and family to get involved in some aspects of cooking, especially on weekends when time is less pressured.
* Plan to eat 'make-ahead' meals or 'almost instant' recipes on your busiest days.
* If it works for your family, a regular cycle of simple, healthy meals served on particular days is fine.
* Enjoy eating meals together as a family at the table as often as you can. This reinforces the important social aspects of food. Try to keep family mealtimes relaxed, and focus conversation on topics other than eating.

Making this eating style work for you and your family

The recipes in this book are based on general healthy eating principles that are appropriate for all members of the family, including:

* sufficient protein-containing foods at each main meal
* eating lots of vegetables
* choosing foods mainly from the core food groups
* minimising consumption of discretionary snack foods.

Therefore the recipes are suitable for all family members, including children and adolescents, although they may need larger or smaller servings depending on their needs and appetite.

Managing hunger

Changing your eating habits can lead to some powerful hunger pangs, especially in the early days as you adjust. The foods listed below contain minimal kilojoules and won't affect your overall energy intake, so they can be added to help manage hunger.

Enjoy them as an extra snack or to boost the volume of your main meals. The spices, herbs and sauces can also be used to boost the flavour and variety of your food and drinks.

> **The recipes in the Vegetable Sides and Soups chapter (page 204) can be enjoyed as low-kilojoule options to accompany main meals, or hunger-busting between-meal snacks.**

Other tips for managing hunger

* Listen to your body's hunger signals – are you really feeling hungry (have a grumble in your tummy), or are you thinking about eating out of boredom or habit?
* Try adding fresh herbs or slices of fruit to plain water, for example: a slice each of lime and lemon; sliced strawberry and a basil leaf; pomegranate seeds and a slice of orange; a slice of cucumber and a few mint leaves.
* Go for a short walk to distract you from the afternoon munchies. Then enjoy a cup of herbal tea.
* If nighttimes are your most common time for snacking, consider whether you can schedule some physical activity or turn your attention to another activity that takes your mind off snacking – talk to a friend, catch up on some chores or have an earlier bedtime.

LOW-KILOJOULE VEGETABLES

asparagus   artichoke   green beans
bean sprouts   bok choy   broccoli
Brussels sprouts   beetroot   carrot
cabbage   capsicum   cauliflower   celery
chilli   chives   choko   corn   cucumber
eggplant   fennel   kale   lettuce
marrow   mushroom   onion
rhubarb   radish   peas   pumpkin
shallot   silverbeet   snowpeas
spinach   swede   tomato
turnip   zucchini

DRINKS

unflavoured mineral water
tea   coffee   herbal teas
cocoa   diet cordial
diet soft drinks

CONDIMENTS

herbs   spices   garlic   ginger   lemon,
vinegar   verjuice   oil-free salad dressing*
mint sauce   wasabi   horseradish   spray oil
mustard   pickles   Vegemite
pickled vegetables (such as cucumbers/capsicum)
tomato sauce*   tomato paste   barbecue sauce*
soy sauce*   fish sauce*   hoisin sauce*
chilli sauce   stock cubes*   clear stocks*
artificial sweeteners   diet topping
diet jelly

* choose salt-reduced versions

Lessons from weight-loss success stories

Changing habits takes a lot of repetition. Habits form because they are the most pleasant and easy option in the short term, but they don't necessarily give us the long-term results we desire. Registers of thousands of people who have successfully maintained significant weight loss show some consistent behaviours and lifestyle choices:

* 78% eat breakfast every day
* 75% weigh themselves at least once a week
* 62% watch less than 10 hours of television each week
* 90% exercise, on average, about 1 hour per day.

We have also spoken to thousands of volunteers over several decades through our clinical research — so we have heard the stories behind the many successes, and of those who didn't reach their goals. Here are some of the 'lessons learned' from the people who have changed their eating habits for the better, and have achieved their goals.

'Break it down'

Set achievable goals by breaking down the 'big hairy audacious' goals into bite-sized chunks. This will help you get some early wins, to build confidence and the motivation to keep going. For example, set 5 kg weight-loss targets, which are achievable and realistic. Once you achieve the first 5 kg target, you can reset to tackle the next 5 kg. A small weight loss (5–10% of body weight) can make a big difference to your health and reduce your risk of developing complications like diabetes, heart disease, stroke and some cancers.

The same principle also applies for changing our eating and physical activity habits, along with the many social and emotional aspects that affect our wellbeing.

'I used to hope for success — now I plan for success'

* Plan your main meals ahead of time. Busy families tend to map out a week in advance, whereas child-free households might only plan a few days ahead. When planning meals, consider household routines: what nights can you enjoy some extra time for meal preparation? What night does dinner need to be pre-made, or super quick to dish up, to avoid resorting to take-aways?
* Double the quantity of a roast or slow-cooked dish and repurpose half for a different meal. (See pages 152 and 178 for meal ideas that can be prepared in bulk and used in a variety of ways.)
* Stick your weekly meal plan on the fridge so everyone can see it and help pitch in.
* Take meat from the freezer the day before and let it thaw in the fridge, so it's ready for cooking the next day.

'If it isn't on my list, it isn't going in my trolley'

Write a shopping list, so your fridge, freezer and pantry are stocked with the right ingredients for healthy meals and snacks. Then follow your list when shopping for groceries, to minimise food wastage and avoid temptation.

'Remove the excuses'

Do a stocktake of the foods in your kitchen, then minimise or remove the tempting 'discretionary' foods. This will be a win for everyone in the family. Keep a good stockpile of frozen vegetables, meats and wholegrain breads in your freezer for those times when shopping time is limited.

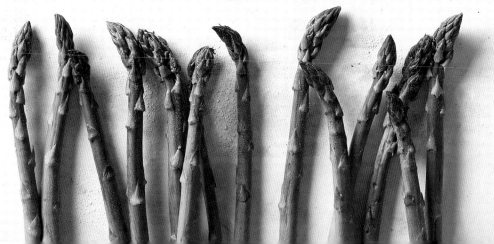

'Batch and dispatch my lunch'

Even though variety is good, developing a new routine — especially for breakfast and lunch — can help a lot. Could you dedicate some time on Sunday evening to prepare a batch of salad jars (page 102–103) for the working week, or simply boil enough eggs for a few days' lunches? Mixing up a batch of overnight oats (page 66) is super quick, and will keep for several days in the fridge for speedy weekday breakfasts.

When the seasons change and a salad isn't satisfying you, switch to a warming soup.

If a recipe makes 4 servings, be sure to divide it up into 4 servings, even if two of those portions are into storage containers in the fridge or freezer, ready for another meal.

'Nothing to see here — just my regular breakfast/lunch routine'

Research shows that the more food variety we are presented with, the more we eat. A fairly tight routine for breakfast and/or lunch shifts focus away from food, and away from the temptation to eat just a little bit extra.

'I know what it tastes like'

Stop and ask yourself: *'Do I really need to eat another piece of chocolate cheesecake?'* Taking a pause can help you gather your resolve not to overeat.

'Portion control: a kilojoule shared is a kilojoule halved'

If you really feel like 'comfort food', make that your indulgence for the week. Eat it slowly, and ask yourself, is it really that good? If it's not — don't finish it.

And cutting your indulgences in half and sharing with someone will enable you to have just a little taste of it, without taking on the full dose of kilojoules.

Do I need protein supplements?

There are a huge variety of protein powders available, with the most common animal-based protein powders being whey and casein from cow's milk, and plant-based options including soy, pea and rice. Generally, obtaining protein from foods is best, though, as foods also contain a variety of other essential vitamins and minerals that we need.

One exception is for people who have a food intolerance or choose a vegetarian or vegan diet. If you can't drink cow's milk, or you choose not to, we recommend replacing it with soy milk due to its protein and calcium content; rice and almond (or other nut) beverages are not protein-equivalent. However, if you follow a vegetarian or vegan diet and choose rice or almond (nut) milks, we suggest adding 1 tablespoon (approx 10 grams) of vegetable-based protein powder per 250 ml of milk.

EMERGING SCIENCE: A role for digital products

Increasingly, weight-loss programs are being delivered online or via smartphone apps. Utilising technology in this way offers a potentially powerful approach for supporting weight loss and encouraging behaviours that are associated with weight-loss success. For example, studies show that self-monitoring is a key behaviour associated with weight-loss success, and technology can make regular self-monitoring more convenient.

There are lots of online tools and apps that help you track your weight and enable you to record what you eat more easily. These tools also allow you to access information almost anywhere, at any time! They have the functionality to enable you to plan menus and create shopping lists, plus they are engaging and fun and provide much-needed support and timely advice. If you are interested in an online weight-management program using higher protein meals, go to totalwellbeingdiet.com.

If you are choosing to boost your protein intake with supplements, look for a product with a high percentage of protein, a complete amino acid profile (all the essential amino acids) and one without additives such as sugars. Check the nutrition panel to compare the amount of protein per 100 grams each product contains.

Protein bars

Protein bars contain varying levels of protein. Many also contain added sugars and fats, making the kilojoule content closer to a meal than a snack. So it's important to take a closer look at what's in them, and consider how they fit into your diet. We recommend aiming for snacks of no more than 400–600 kJ.

Protein powders

As mentioned, most protein powders consist of soy, pea or dairy (whey or casein) proteins. These powders may also contain several other ingredients, such as vegetable gums, thickeners, artificial sweeteners, artificial flavours and indigestible fibres (inulin). Check the nutrition panels of different products to compare how much protein each 100 grams contains.

Meal replacement shakes

Meal replacements, as the name suggests, are designed to replace a whole meal. As such they are higher in kilojoules and usually contain a combination of carbohydrates, proteins and fats along with an array of vitamins and minerals. The protein levels vary, so if you do choose one of these, higher-protein options are a better choice — although few contain 25 grams of protein per serve.

Impromy™ (impromy.com) is a higher-protein, partial-meal replacement program, in which one or more meals are replaced with shakes. It was developed in collaboration with CSIRO and offers support from trained pharmacy staff.

Skim milk powder

Dried skim milk powder is an inexpensive high-quality protein source that contains both casein and whey proteins. Each 100 grams of skim milk powder provides 36 grams of protein and 1455 kilojoules.

It also contains lactose, a naturally occurring dairy sugar, so it is not suitable for people who are lactose-intolerant or have a dairy allergy.

Q: What happens if I have too much protein?

A: We know that people with a higher lean muscle mass, and those doing high levels of resistance exercise, require a higher dietary protein intake. However, if you eat too many kilojoules from protein and don't cut back on kilojoules from other foods (i.e. carbohydrates, fats and alcohol), you will gain weight. When you eat more protein than your body needs, the excess protein is converted by your body to energy. This is either used or stored as body fat.

There has been concern that a very high protein intake may place extra stress on the kidneys. However, research suggests this is only the case for individuals with pre-existing poor kidney function or disease. In the sample meal plans provided in this book, as in our online programs, the total amount of protein provided is similar to that of the typical Australian diet – about 80–100 grams per day – and research suggests there are no detrimental health effects associated with this level of protein intake. Nevertheless, when embarking on changes to your diet and lifestyle it is always recommended that you consult your healthcare team. This is particularly important if you have poor kidney function, or suffer from type 2 diabetes (a condition that increases the risk of poor kidney health).

PART THREE

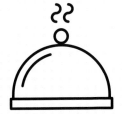

The Recipes

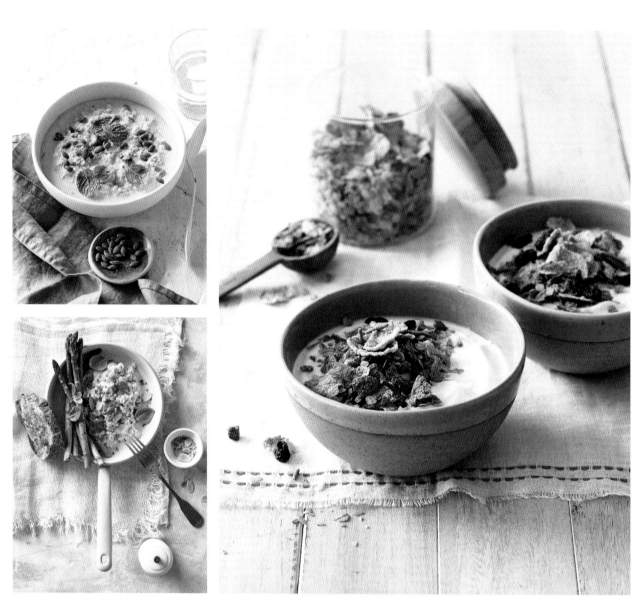

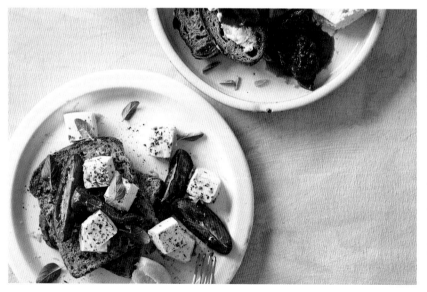

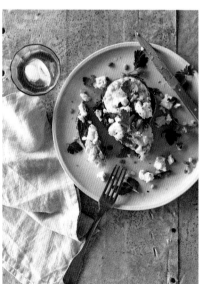

1. Breakfast

Porridge with honey-nut crunch and mocha

Preparation: 10 minutes, plus cooling time ✳ **Cooking:** 15 minutes
Difficulty: Medium

A

SERVES 4

28 g slivered almonds, roughly chopped
1 teaspoon honey, warmed (see Notes),
    plus 1 teaspoon extra
¼ teaspoon ground cinnamon
60 g Sultana Bran, roughly crushed
1½ cups (135 g) rolled oats
2 litres low-fat milk
1 tablespoon instant coffee granules
1 tablespoon cocoa powder

Preheat the oven to 200°C (180°C fan-forced). Line a baking tray with baking paper.

Spread the chopped almonds over the prepared baking tray (keep them close together but in a single layer), drizzle evenly with the warmed honey and sprinkle with cinnamon. Bake for 10–12 minutes or until golden. Remove from the oven and leave to cool on the tray, then break into small pieces. Place in a bowl with the Sultana Bran and toss to combine.

Meanwhile, place the oats and 1 litre of the milk in a large saucepan over low–medium heat. Bring to a gentle simmer, stirring constantly, then reduce the heat to low and cook, stirring occasionally, for 15 minutes or until the oats are soft and the mixture has thickened.

Shortly before the oats are ready, combine the coffee, cocoa powder, extra honey and remaining milk in a separate saucepan over low–medium heat. Whisk constantly until the coffee and cocoa have dissolved and the mixture is smooth, then continue to whisk until the mixture comes to a simmer. Remove the pan from the heat and cover to keep warm.

Divide the oats among serving bowls and sprinkle with the nut mixture. Pour the warm mocha into mugs and serve alongside.

NOTES

Warming the honey makes it easier to drizzle. You can either heat it in the microwave on high for a few seconds or place it in a small heatproof jug and pop the jug in a bowl of boiling water for a minute or so.

You can easily make a double batch of this recipe. Store the cooled nut clusters in an airtight container at room temperature and the oats and mocha in separate airtight containers in the fridge. All the elements will keep for up to 3 days. Reheat the oats and mocha either on the stovetop over low heat or separately in the microwave.

Increase or decrease the quantities of coffee and cocoa to suit your taste.

UNITS PER SERVE Grains **2** ✳ Meat and alternatives **0** ✳ Fruit **0** ✳ Vegetables **0** ✳ Dairy **2** ✳ Fats and oils **1**

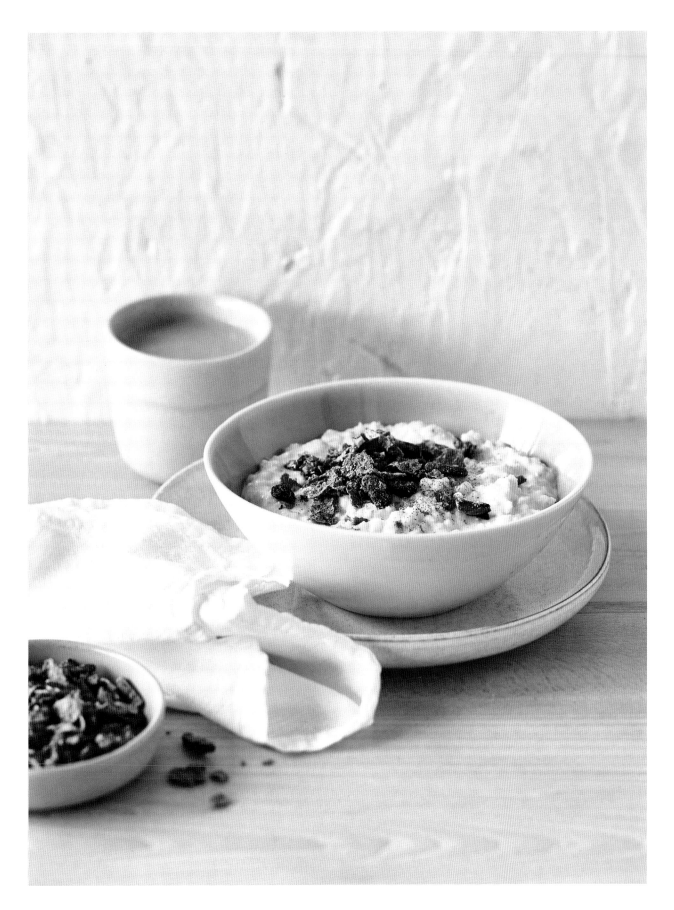

BREAKFAST SMOOTHIES

A

All recipes serve 1

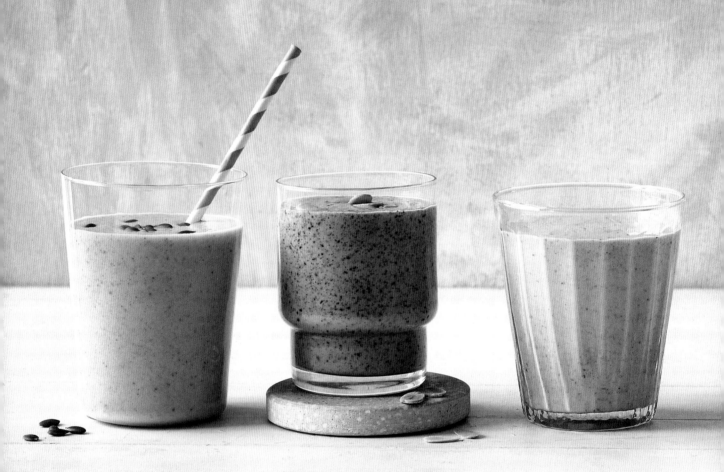

High-fibre pear

Blend together 1 cored pear,
60 g high-fibre cereal and 2 cups
(500 ml) low-fat milk. Serve topped
with 7 g pumpkin seeds (pepitas).

UNITS PER SERVE

Grains **2** ✽ Meat and alternatives **0**
Fruit **1** ✽ Vegetables **0** ✽ Dairy **2**
Fats and oils **1**

Berry bran

Blend together 150 g mixed fresh
or frozen berries, 60 g Sultana Bran
cereal and 2 cups (500 ml) low-fat
milk. Serve topped with 7 g toasted
flaked almonds.

UNITS PER SERVE

Grains **2** ✽ Meat and alternatives **0**
Fruit **1** ✽ Vegetables **0** ✽ Dairy **2**
Fats and oils **1**

Hunger buster banana

Blend together 1 banana, ½ cup (45 g)
quick oats, 200 g low-fat vanilla
yoghurt, 1 cup (250 ml) low-fat milk
and 20 g avocado.

UNITS PER SERVE

Grains **2** ✽ Meat and alternatives **0**
Fruit **1** ✽ Vegetables **0** ✽ Dairy **2**
Fats and oils **1**

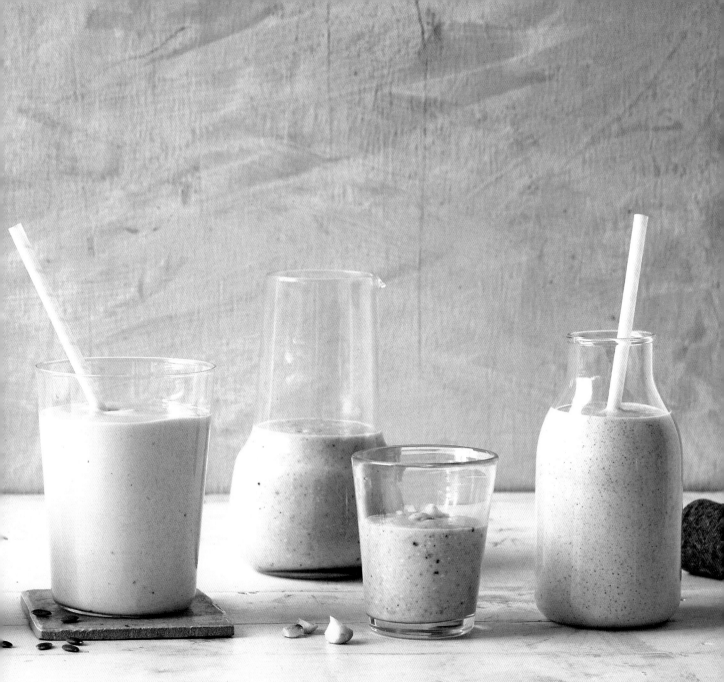

Passion protein

Blend together the seeds and juice of 2 passionfruit, 60 g protein-rich wheat cereal flakes, 120 g fresh reduced-fat ricotta, 1 cup (250 ml) low-fat milk and 7 g chopped raw almonds.

UNITS PER SERVE
Grains **2** ✳ Meat and alternatives **0**
Fruit **0.5** ✳ Vegetables **0** ✳ Dairy **2**
Fats and oils **1**

Muesli maca mango

Blend together the flesh of ½ large mango, 60 g natural muesli and 2 cups (500 ml) low-fat milk. Serve topped with 7 g toasted, chopped unsalted macadamias.

UNITS PER SERVE
Grains **2** ✳ Meat and alternatives **0**
Fruit **1** ✳ Vegetables **0** ✳ Dairy **2**
Fats and oils **1**

Apple pie oats

Blend together ⅓ cup (80 g) unsweetened apple puree, ½ cup (45 g) quick oats, 7 g almonds, ½ teaspoon ground cinnamon, 200 g low-fat vanilla yoghurt and 1 cup (250 ml) low-fat milk.

UNITS PER SERVE
Grains **2** ✳ Meat and alternatives **0**
Fruit **0.5** ✳ Vegetables **0** ✳ Dairy **2**
Fats and oils **1**

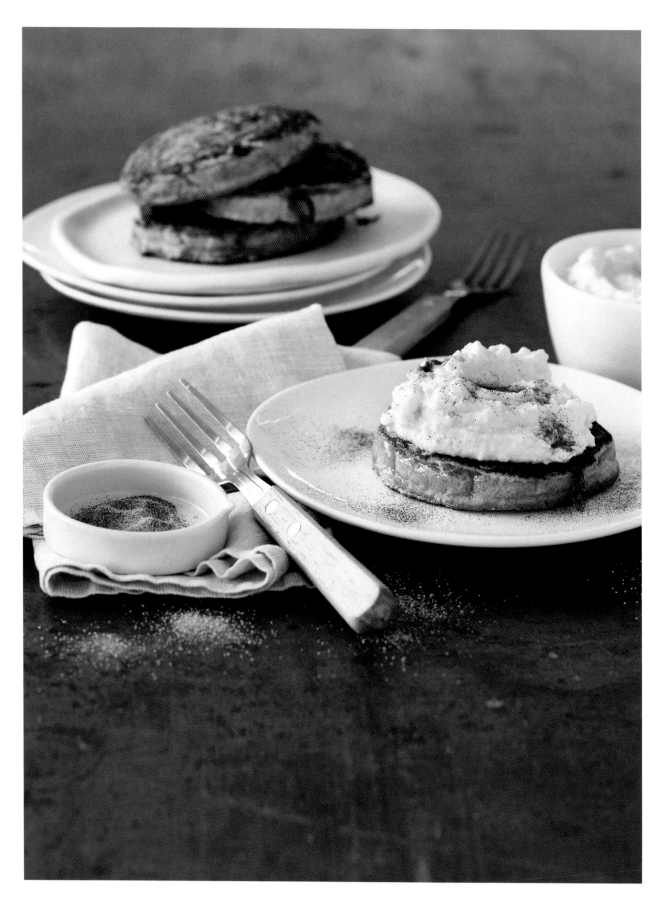

Frenched crumpets with ricotta cream

Preparation: 15 minutes, plus standing time ✳ **Cooking:** 5 minutes
Difficulty: Easy

B

SERVES 4

8 large eggs
1 teaspoon vanilla
4 x 60 g wholemeal crumpets
2 tablespoons light margarine
300 g fresh reduced-fat ricotta
300 g low-fat vanilla dairy dessert
    (e.g. Fruche fromage frais)
2 teaspoons caster sugar
½ teaspoon ground cinnamon

Place the eggs and vanilla in a flat dish and whisk together with a fork. Add the crumpets to the egg mixture and turn to coat well on both sides. Stand, turning occasionally, for 15 minutes or until the crumpets have absorbed the egg mixture.

Melt the margarine in a large non-stick frying pan over low–medium heat. Add the crumpets and cook for 2–3 minutes each side or until cooked and golden.

Meanwhile, using a whisk or a hand-held electric mixer, beat the ricotta and dairy dessert together until smooth and light.

Combine the sugar and cinnamon in a small bowl.

Top the hot crumpets with the ricotta cream and sprinkle with cinnamon sugar. Serve warm.

NOTES

You'll need 2 x 150 g tubs of vanilla dairy dessert for this recipe. Store the leftover ricotta cream in an airtight container in the fridge for up to 3 days.

UNITS PER SERVE Grains **1** ✳ Meat and alternatives **1** ✳ Fruit **0** ✳ Vegetables **0** ✳ Dairy **1** ✳ Fats and oils **1**

Sweet spiced oats

Preparation: 15 minutes, plus overnight resting time ✳ **Cooking:** nil
Difficulty: Easy

A

SERVES 4

2 cups (180 g) quick oats
3 cups (750 ml) low-fat milk
1 kg low-fat vanilla or strawberry yoghurt
28 g pumpkin seeds (pepitas),
   lightly toasted
½ teaspoon brown sugar
½ teaspoon ground ginger
mint leaves (optional)

Combine the oats, milk and 200 g of the yoghurt in a large bowl. Cover tightly and store in the fridge overnight.

The next day, divide the remaining yoghurt among serving bowls and top with the oat mixture.

Combine the pumpkin seeds, sugar and ginger and sprinkle over the oat mixture. Top with mint leaves, if desired.

NOTES

You can easily make a double or triple batch of the overnight oats up to the end of step 1. Store in an airtight container in the fridge for up to 4 days.

Any type of low-fat yoghurt is delicious in this recipe so use what you have. You can swap the ground ginger for mixed spice or ground cinnamon, if desired.

UNITS PER SERVE Grains **2** ✳ Meat and alternatives **0** ✳ Fruit **0** ✳ Vegetables **0** ✳ Dairy **2** ✳ Fats and oils **1**

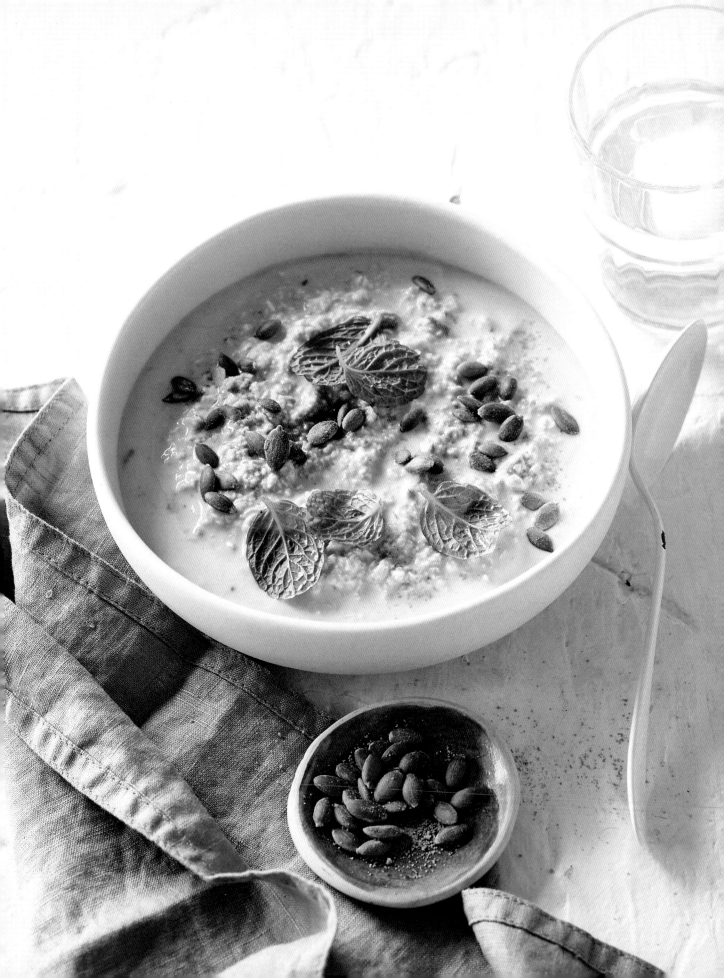

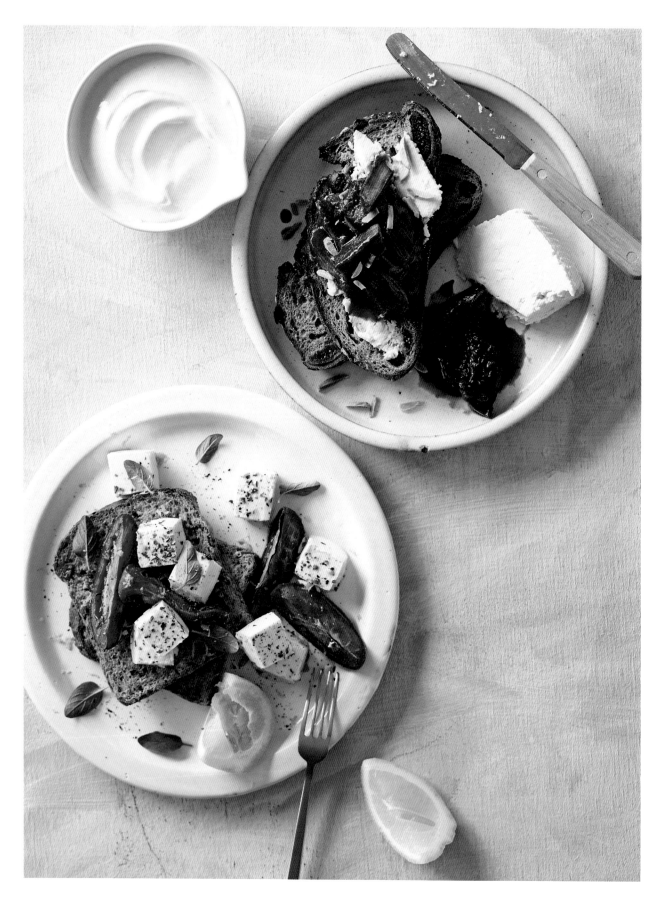

Rhubarb and ricotta fruit toast

Preparation: 10 minutes, plus resting time
Cooking: 10 minutes
Difficulty: Easy

A

SERVES 4

2 tablespoons diet, no-sugar apple and raspberry cordial
1 bunch rhubarb, trimmed and cut into 4 cm lengths
   (see Notes)
8 x 40 g slices wholemeal sourdough fruit loaf
480 g fresh reduced-fat ricotta
28 g slivered almonds, toasted
800 g low-fat vanilla yoghurt

Place the cordial, three-quarters of the rhubarb and 2 tablespoons water in a small saucepan over low–medium heat. Cook, stirring occasionally, for 3–5 minutes or until the rhubarb has softened. Add the remaining rhubarb and cook for 30 seconds. Remove the pan from the heat and stand, covered, for 2 minutes.

Chargrill or grill the fruit loaf for 1–2 minutes each side until golden.

Spread a wedge of ricotta over each hot slice of toast, then spoon over the warm rhubarb mixture. Sprinkle with the almonds and serve with the yoghurt alongside.

NOTES

The rhubarb in this recipe comes from your 'anytime' fruit units. You can easily make a double or triple batch of the rhubarb mixture up to the end of step 1, then store in an airtight container in the fridge for up to 4 days.

In the summer months, use berries instead. Cook 300 g berries with the cordial and water for 3 minutes.

UNITS PER SERVE Grains **2** ✳ Meat and alternatives **0**
Fruit **0.5** ✳ Vegetables **0** ✳ Dairy **2** ✳ Fats and oils **1**

Grilled Italian feta and tomatoes on toast

Preparation: 15 minutes
Cooking: 5 minutes
Difficulty: Easy

A

SERVES 4

4 tomatoes, quartered lengthways
640 g feta, cut into 2 cm pieces (see Notes)
1 teaspoon dried Italian mixed herbs
1 tablespoon olive oil
1 lemon, zest finely grated and lemon cut into wedges
¼ cup oregano leaves
8 x 40 g slices wholegrain bread, toasted

Preheat the oven grill to high. Place the tomato, cut-side up, on a non-stick baking tray and grill for 1 minute.

Add the feta to the tray and sprinkle evenly with the dried herbs. Drizzle over the olive oil and season to taste with freshly ground black pepper. Grill for 4 minutes or until light golden. Remove from the grill and sprinkle with the lemon zest and oregano.

Divide the toast among serving plates and top with the feta and tomato. Serve warm with lemon wedges.

NOTES

If you want to reduce the salt content of the feta, cut it into cubes and place in a bowl of water for 30 minutes to steep. Drain before use.

UNITS PER SERVE Grains **2** ✳ Meat and alternatives **0**
Fruit **0** ✳ Vegetables **1** ✳ Dairy **2** ✳ Fats and oils **1**

EASY EGGS ON TOAST

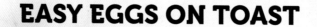

B

All recipes serve 1, and include a 40 g slice of multigrain toast.

Soft-boiled with zesty spinach

Soft-boil 2 large eggs, then peel and halve lengthways. Meanwhile, heat 1 teaspoon olive oil in a small frying pan over medium heat, add 1 cup (30 g) baby spinach leaves and cook for 1 minute or until just wilted. Remove the pan from the heat and stir through ¼ cup small basil leaves and the finely grated zest and juice of ½ small lemon. Season to taste with freshly ground black pepper. Serve warm on toast with the soft-boiled eggs, sprinkled with ½ cup (40 g) grated parmesan.

UNITS PER SERVE
Grains **1** ✻ Meat and alternatives **1**
Fruit **0** ✻ Vegetables **1** ✻ Dairy **1**
Fats and oils **1**

Hard-boiled with zucchini slaw

Hard-boil 2 large eggs, then peel and slice. Meanwhile, grate 1 small zucchini and combine in a bowl with 80 g feta, 1 thinly sliced spring onion (white and green parts), 2 teaspoons white wine vinegar and ½ teaspoon wholegrain mustard. Season to taste with freshly ground black pepper. Serve on toast with the hard-boiled eggs, sprinkled with 7 g toasted slivered almonds and mint.

UNITS PER SERVE
Grains **1** ✻ Meat and alternatives **1**
Fruit **0** ✻ Vegetables **1.5** ✻ Dairy **1**
Fats and oils **1**

Fried with paprika veggies

Melt 2 teaspoons light margarine in a small saucepan over medium heat. Add 2 teaspoons sweet paprika, ½ sliced onion and 1 sliced and seeded small red capsicum and cook for 5 minutes or until very soft. Meanwhile, lightly spray a non-stick frying pan with light olive oil and pan-fry 2 large eggs over medium–high heat for 2 minutes or until the whites are set and crispy around the edges and the yolks are still soft. Spread 120 g fresh reduced-fat ricotta over the toast. Top with the vegetable mixture, then the eggs and sprinkle with flat-leaf parsley.

UNITS PER SERVE
Grains **1** ✻ Meat and alternatives **1**
Fruit **0** ✻ Vegetables **3** ✻ Dairy **1**
Fats and oils **1**

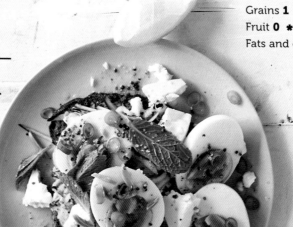

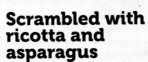

Scrambled in a mushroom cup

Preheat the oven grill to high. Grill 1 large field mushroom for 5 minutes, turning once. Place on the toast on a serving plate and fill with 40 g crumbled cheddar. Meanwhile, scramble 2 large eggs, 1 small crushed garlic clove and 2 teaspoons thyme leaves in a small non-stick frying pan over medium heat for 2 minutes or until the egg is just set. Spoon the scrambled egg over the cheddar in the mushroom cup. Top with ⅔ cup (20 g) baby rocket leaves and 7 g toasted pine nuts.

UNITS PER SERVE

Grains **1** ✳ Meat and alternatives **1**
Fruit **0** ✳ Vegetables **1.5** ✳ Dairy **1**
Fats and oils **1**

Scrambled with ricotta and asparagus

Melt 2 teaspoons light margarine in a non-stick frying pan over medium–high heat. Trim 1 bunch of thin asparagus spears and halve them crossways, then add to the pan and cook for 1 minute. Whisk together 2 large eggs and 120 g fresh reduced-fat ricotta, add to the asparagus and cook, stirring occasionally, for 2 minutes or until the egg is just set. Spoon the egg mixture over the toast and season to taste with freshly ground black pepper. Sprinkle with 1 tablespoon dill and serve.

UNITS PER SERVE

Grains **1** ✳ Meat and alternatives **1**
Fruit **0** ✳ Vegetables **1** ✳ Dairy **1**
Fats and oils **1**

Poached with tomato salsa

Poach 2 large eggs to your liking. Spread 120 g reduced-fat cottage cheese over the toast. Add 20 g avocado, 1 finely chopped tomato, 1 tablespoon finely chopped chives and 2 teaspoons balsamic vinegar. Top with the eggs, season with freshly ground black pepper and serve.

UNITS PER SERVE

Grains **1** ✳ Meat and alternatives **1**
Fruit **0** ✳ Vegetables **1.5** ✳ Dairy **1**
Fats and oils **1**

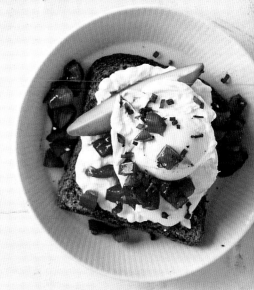

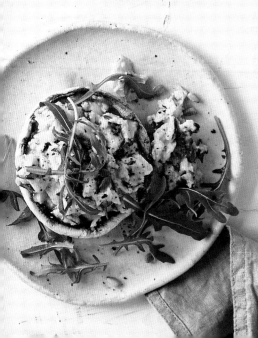

Fruit toast bake

Preparation: 20 minutes, plus standing time ✳ **Cooking:** 1 hour 5 minutes
Difficulty: Medium

B

SERVES 4

2 tablespoons light margarine
4 x 40 g slices fruit loaf
8 large eggs
400 g low-fat vanilla custard
½ teaspoon ground cinnamon
400 g low-fat vanilla yoghurt

Preheat the oven to 180°C (160°C fan-forced). Using 1 teaspoon of the margarine, grease an 18 cm round baking dish.

Spread the remaining margarine over the fruit loaf slices, then cut each slice into four triangles.

Whisk the eggs, custard and cinnamon in a bowl until smooth and well combined. Carefully pour the mixture into the prepared dish. Add the fruit toast triangles, one at a time, submerging each piece into the egg mixture to coat on both sides before adding the next. Stand for 15 minutes, turning and re-submerging the fruit loaf pieces occasionally, until the egg mixture has been completely absorbed.

Loosely cover the dish with a tented piece of foil (you don't want it to touch the bread). Bake for 50 minutes, then remove the foil and bake for a further 15 minutes or until cooked and golden.

Serve warm with vanilla yoghurt.

NOTES

This is a great option for a leisurely weekend breakfast due to its longer cooking time.

UNITS PER SERVE Grains **1** ✳ Meat and alternatives **1** ✳ Fruit **0** ✳ Vegetables **0** ✳ Dairy **1** ✳ Fats and oils **1**

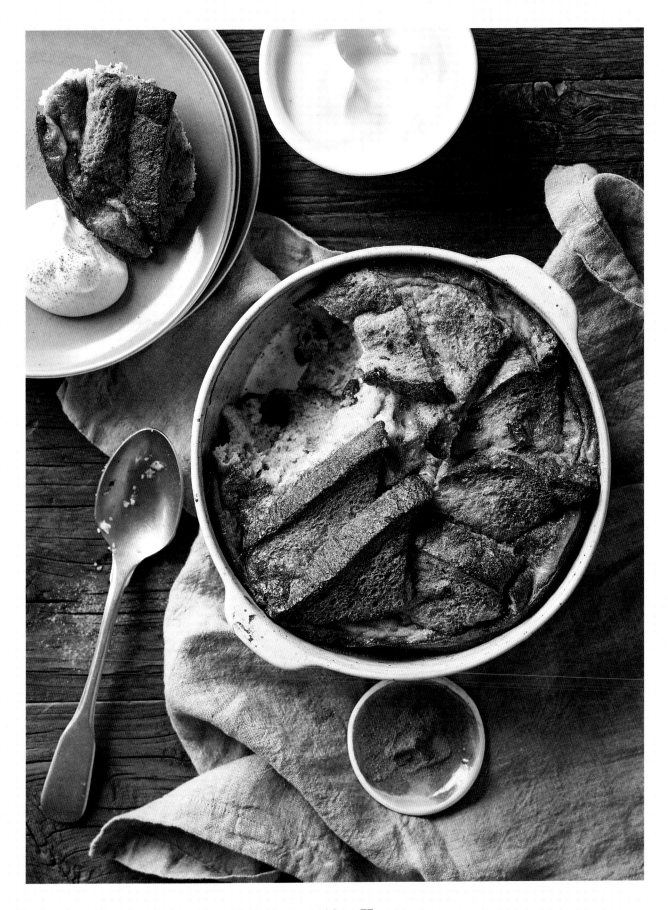

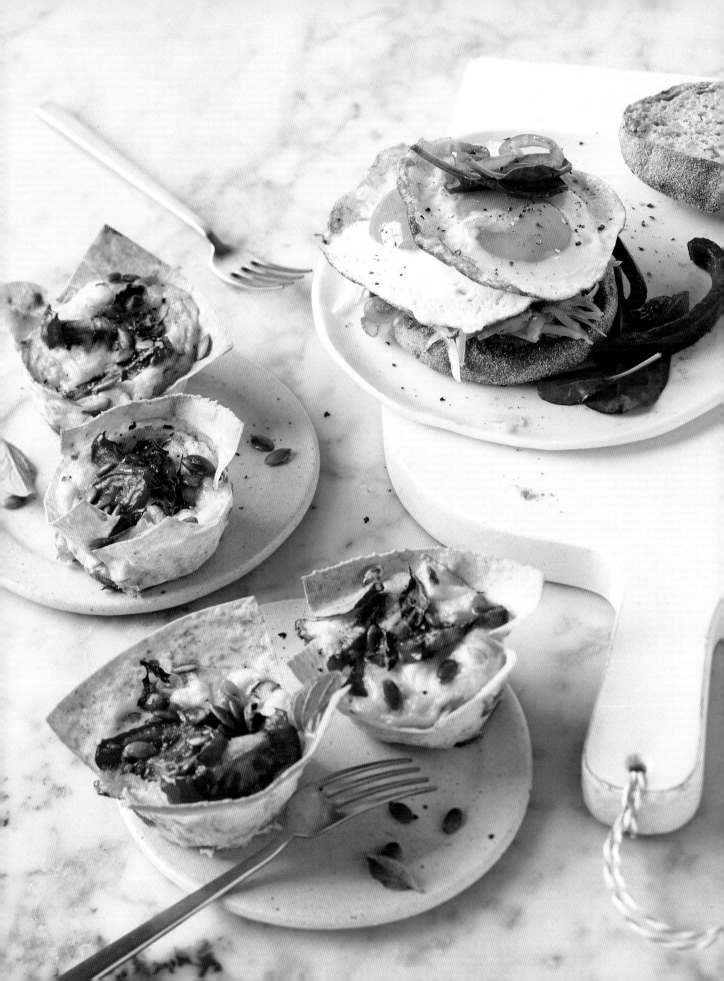

Double egg and vegetable muffins

Preparation: 15 minutes
Cooking: 10 minutes
Difficulty: Medium

B

SERVES 4

2 tablespoons light margarine
1 onion, thinly sliced into rings
1 small red capsicum, seeded and sliced
50 g baby spinach leaves
1 tablespoon salt-reduced barbecue sauce
light olive oil spray, for cooking
8 large eggs
4 x 60 g wholemeal English muffins, split and toasted
160 g tasty cheese, coarsely grated

Melt the margarine in a medium saucepan over medium heat. Add the onion and capsicum and cook, stirring occasionally, for 5 minutes or until cooked and golden. Add the spinach, barbecue sauce and 2 tablespoons water and cook, tossing, for 2 minutes or until the spinach has wilted. Season with freshly ground black pepper.

Meanwhile, lightly spray a large non-stick frying pan with olive oil and heat over medium–high heat. Crack the eggs into the pan and cook for 2–3 minutes or until the whites are set and crisp around the edges and the yolks are still runny. (Use two frying pans if you don't have one large enough to hold eight eggs.)

Divide the toasted muffins among serving plates. Top one half with cheese, the hot vegetable mixture and the fried eggs, then top with the other muffin half. Serve hot.

UNITS PER SERVE Grains **1** ✳ Meat and alternatives **1**
Fruit **0** ✳ Vegetables **1** ✳ Dairy **1** ✳ Fats and oils **1**

Ricotta breakfast quiches

Preparation: 20 minutes, plus resting time
Cooking: 35 minutes
Difficulty: Medium

B

SERVES 4

light olive oil spray, for cooking
8 x 25 g wholemeal or rye mountain breads
8 large eggs
240 g fresh reduced-fat ricotta
80 g cheddar, grated
2 teaspoons finely grated lemon zest
2 spring onions, white and green parts thinly sliced
¼ cup oregano leaves
1 large tomato, thinly sliced
28 g pumpkin seeds (pepitas)

Preheat the oven to 200°C (180°C fan-forced). Lightly spray eight holes of a non-stick 12-hole, ⅓ cup muffin tin with olive oil. Cut each mountain bread into four pieces, then layer four pieces of the bread into each of the prepared holes, making sure that the base and side are evenly covered. Lightly spray with olive oil.

Combine the eggs, ricotta, cheddar, lemon zest and spring onion in a large bowl and season with freshly ground black pepper. Spoon the mixture evenly into the bread-lined muffin holes. Sprinkle with oregano, top with tomato and lightly spray with the oil.

Bake for 25 minutes, then sprinkle with the pumpkin seeds and bake for a further 8–10 minutes or until golden and set in the middle when tested with a skewer. Rest in the tin for 3 minutes, then serve warm.

UNITS PER SERVE Grains **1** ✳ Meat and alternatives **1**
Fruit **0** ✳ Vegetables **0.5** ✳ Dairy **1** ✳ Fats and oils **1**

Toasted muesli bowls

Preparation: 10 minutes, plus cooling time * **Cooking:** 25 minutes
Difficulty: Easy

A

SERVES 4

1 tablespoon sunflower oil
1 cup (120 g) 97% fat-free natural muesli
½ teaspoon mixed spice
⅔ cup (60 g) Sultana Bran
1⅓ cups (60 g) wheat cereal flakes
1.6 kg low-fat vanilla or apricot yoghurt

Preheat the oven to 180°C (160°C fan-forced). Line a large baking tray with baking paper.

Combine the sunflower oil, muesli and mixed spice in a bowl, then spread evenly over the prepared tray. Bake for 20–25 minutes, tossing occasionally, until golden. Remove from the oven and cool completely on the tray.

Combine the cooled muesli mixture, Sultana Bran and wheat flakes in a bowl. Divide the yoghurt among serving bowls and level the surface. Top with the muesli mixture and serve.

NOTES

You can easily make a double or triple batch of the muesli mixture up to the end of step 1. Store in an airtight container at room temperature for up to 2 weeks.

UNITS PER SERVE Grains **2** * Meat and alternatives **0** * Fruit **0** * Vegetables **0** * Dairy **2** * Fats and oils **1**

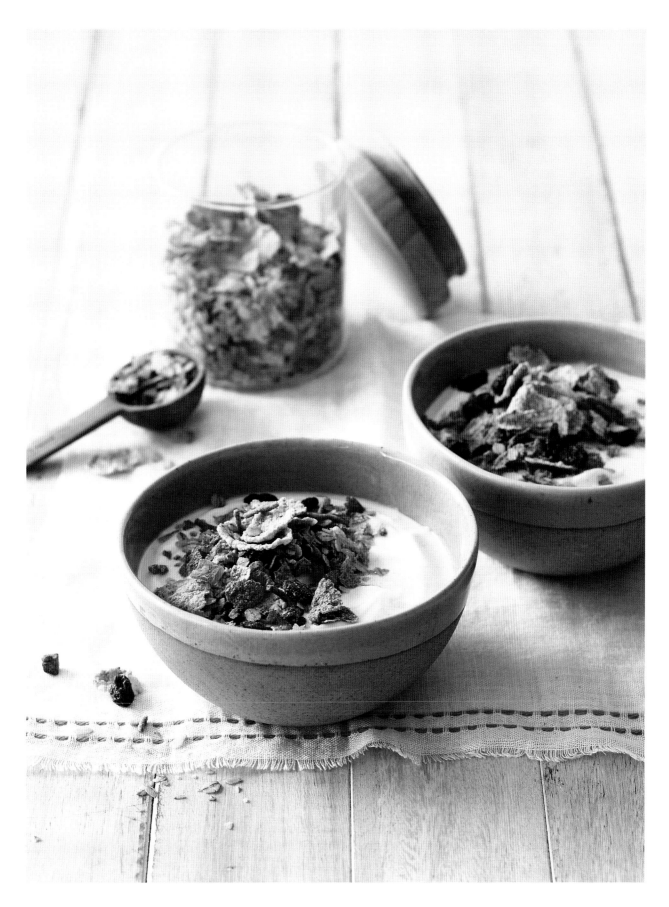

Baked ricotta with seasonal veg

Preparation: 20 minutes, plus resting time * **Cooking:** 35 minutes
Difficulty: Easy

A

SERVES 4

480 g fresh reduced-fat ricotta
120 g cheddar, coarsely grated
200 g low-fat natural Greek-style yoghurt
¼ cup chopped chives
2 tablespoons thyme leaves
1 teaspoon freshly ground black pepper
light olive oil spray, for cooking
100 g button mushrooms
1 small red capsicum, seeded and sliced
1 small red onion, cut into wedges
250 g cherry tomatoes
1 tablespoon rosemary leaves, chopped
1 tablespoon olive oil
20 g baby rocket leaves
8 x 40 g slices multigrain bread, toasted

Preheat the oven to 200°C (180°C fan-forced). Line the base and side of a 20 cm square cake tin and a large baking tray with baking paper.

Combine the ricotta, cheddar, yoghurt, chives, thyme and pepper in a bowl. Press the mixture firmly into the prepared cake tin and level the surface. Lightly spray the top with olive oil and bake for 15 minutes.

Spread out the mushrooms, capsicum, onion, tomatoes and rosemary on the prepared baking tray and add the olive oil. Season with freshly ground black pepper. Add to the oven with the ricotta mixture and bake them both for a further 20 minutes or until the ricotta is firm and golden, and the vegetables are cooked. Remove from the oven and allow the ricotta to rest in the tin for 5 minutes before cutting. Toss the rocket through the vegetables on the tray.

Cut the baked ricotta into pieces and serve warm with the baked vegetables and toast.

UNITS PER SERVE Grains **2** * Meat and alternatives **0** * Fruit **0** * Vegetables **2** * Dairy **2** * Fats and oils **1**

Smoked salmon toasts

Preparation: 15 minutes ✳ **Cooking:** 5 minutes
Difficulty: Easy

— B —

SERVES 4

100 g low-fat natural Greek-style yoghurt
1 small lemon, zest finely grated,
    lemon cut into wedges
1 tablespoon baby capers in brine,
    rinsed and chopped
2 spring onions, white and green
    parts thinly sliced
2 tablespoons dill
4 x 40 g slices sourdough
light olive oil spray, for cooking
1 clove garlic, halved
1 bunch rocket, leaves trimmed
80 g avocado, sliced
400 g smoked salmon slices
140 g parmesan, shaved

Combine the yoghurt, lemon zest, capers, spring onion and dill in a bowl and season with freshly ground black pepper.

Heat a large chargrill pan over high heat.

Lightly spray both sides of the bread slices with olive oil. Chargrill for 1 minute on each side until golden. Remove and immediately rub the hot toast with the cut sides of the garlic clove. Divide among serving plates.

Top the toasts with rocket, avocado and salmon slices, drizzle with the yoghurt mixture and sprinkle with parmesan. Serve with lemon wedges.

NOTES

If you can't find whole bunches of rocket, use 2 cups (120 g) small rocket leaves instead.

UNITS PER SERVE Grains **1** ✳ Meat and alternatives **1** ✳ Fruit **0** ✳ Vegetables **0.5** ✳ Dairy **1** ✳ Fats and oils **1**

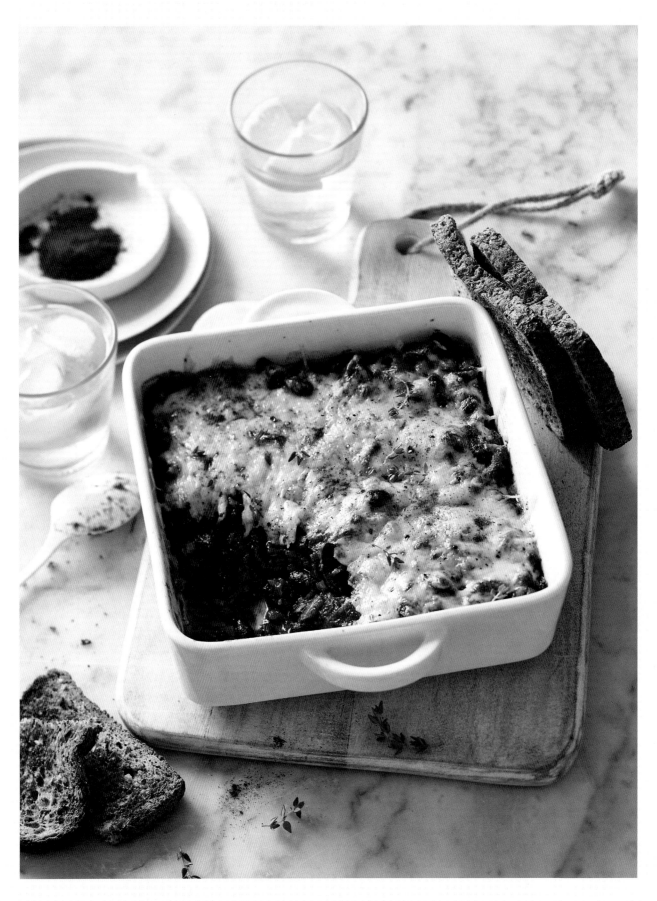

Cheesy breakfast beans

Preparation: 15 minutes ✽ **Cooking:** 25 minutes
Difficulty: Medium

B

SERVES 4

1 tablespoon olive oil
1 onion, finely chopped
2 teaspoons sweet paprika
1 x 400 g tin crushed tomatoes
600 g drained and rinsed tinned red
    kidney beans (see Notes)
160 g tasty cheese, coarsely grated
½ teaspoon dried mixed herbs
4 x 40 g slices multigrain bread,
    toasted, halved

Heat the olive oil in a large saucepan over medium heat. Add the onion and paprika and cook, stirring occasionally, for 5 minutes or until softened and light golden.

Reduce the heat to low. Add the tomatoes and kidney beans and cook, stirring occasionally, for 15 minutes or until the mixture has reduced and thickened slightly.

Preheat the oven grill to high.

Transfer the bean mixture to a 1 litre flameproof baking dish. Sprinkle over the cheese and then the mixed herbs. Cook under the grill for 2–3 minutes or until the cheese is melted and bubbling. Season with freshly ground black pepper.

Serve the beans hot with toast for dipping.

NOTES

Because you will be draining off quite a bit of liquid, you will need to buy three 400 g tins of beans to have the required quantity for this recipe. Store the leftover beans in an airtight container in the fridge for up to 3 days or freeze in an airtight container for up to 3 months.

UNITS PER SERVE Grains **1** ✽ Meat and alternatives **1** ✽ Fruit **0** ✽ Vegetables **1.5** ✽ Dairy **1** ✽ Fats and oils **1**

Creamy vanilla rice

Preparation: 10 minutes ❄ **Cooking:** 45 minutes
Difficulty: Easy

A

SERVES 4

2 litres low-fat milk

2 teaspoons vanilla

1.5 cups (320 g) medium-grain white rice

1 tablespoon finely grated orange zest

28 g unsalted macadamias, toasted
  and finely chopped

Combine the milk and vanilla in a large saucepan over medium heat and bring to a simmer. Stir in the rice, then reduce the heat to low and cook, partially covered and stirring occasionally, for 40–45 minutes or until the rice is tender and the mixture has thickened.

Divide among serving bowls and top with the orange zest and macadamia. Serve warm.

UNITS PER SERVE Grains **2** ❄ Meat and alternatives **0** ❄ Fruit **0** ❄ Vegetables **0** ❄ Dairy **2** ❄ Fats and oils **1**

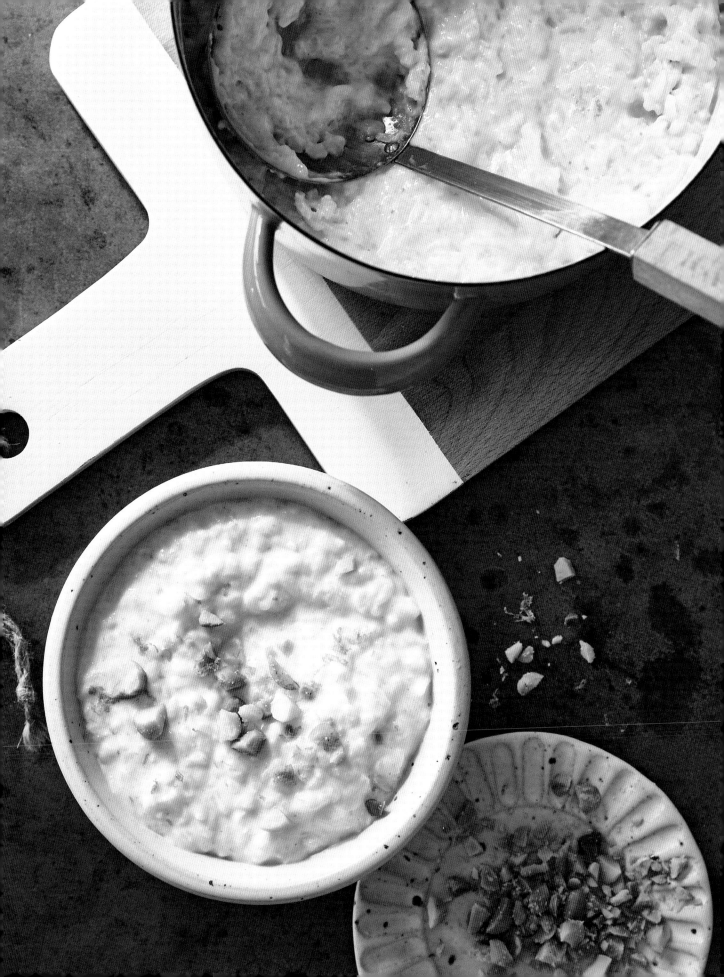

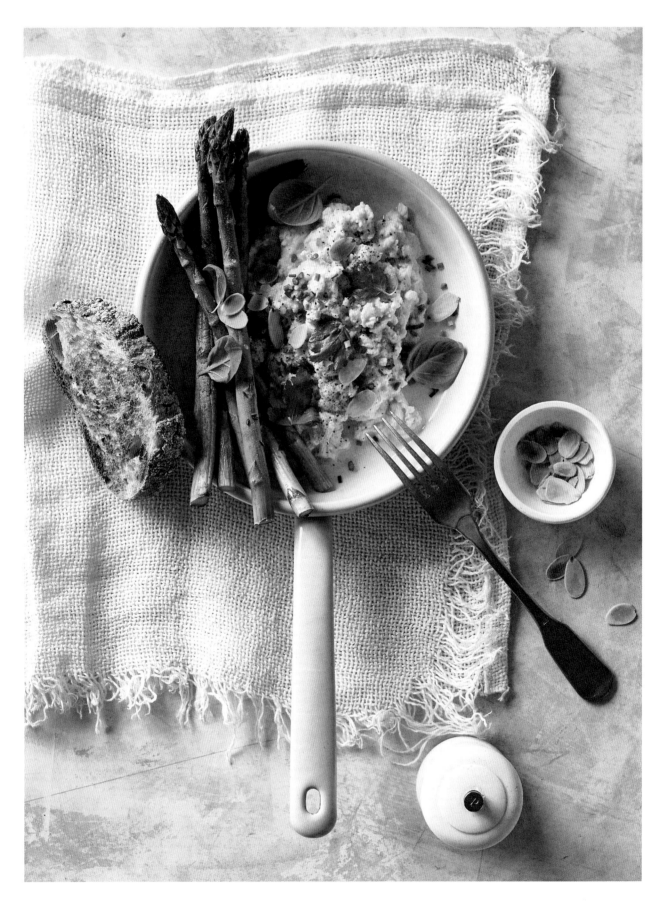

Cheesy scramble with asparagus

Preparation: 15 minutes ✳ **Cooking:** 6 minutes
Difficulty: Easy

— B —

SERVES 4

light olive oil spray, for cooking
8 large eggs
480 g reduced-fat cottage cheese
2 bunches asparagus, trimmed
28 g flaked almonds
1 teaspoon cumin seeds
½ cup flat-leaf parsley leaves
½ cup small basil leaves
1 tablespoon finely chopped chives
4 x 40 g slices multigrain bread, toasted

Lightly spray a large non-stick frying pan with olive oil and heat over medium heat. Preheat the oven grill to high.

Place the eggs and cottage cheese in a large bowl and whisk with a fork. Season with freshly ground black pepper. Add to the frying pan and cook, gently stirring occasionally, for 3 minutes or until the egg is softly set.

Meanwhile, place the asparagus on a non-stick baking tray and lightly spray with olive oil. Cook under the grill for 1 minute. Turn over and sprinkle with the almonds and cumin seeds, then spray with a little more oil and return to the grill for a further 2 minutes or until just tender and golden.

Divide the scrambled egg and asparagus among serving plates and sprinkle with the parsley, basil and chives. Serve warm with toast.

UNITS PER SERVE Grains **1** ✳ Meat and alternatives **1** ✳ Fruit **0** ✳ Vegetables **0.5** ✳ Dairy **1** ✳ Fats and oils **1**

Breakfast **85**

Avocado melts

Preparation: 15 minutes * **Cooking:** 5 minutes
Difficulty: Easy

A

SERVES 4

½ (80 g) medium-sized avocado

3 teaspoons red wine vinegar

2 spring onions, white and green
    parts thinly sliced

2 tablespoons finely chopped basil,
    plus extra small leaves to serve

8 x 40 g slices wholegrain
    crusty sourdough

320 g tasty cheese, cut into 8 slices

Preheat the oven grill to high.

Mash the avocado, vinegar, spring onion and chopped basil in a bowl and season to taste with freshly ground black pepper. Set aside.

Place the sourdough slices on a non-stick baking tray and grill for 1–2 minutes or until golden. Turn them over and top with the cheese slices. Grill for another 1–2 minutes or until the cheese is melted and bubbling.

Immediately top four of the cheese toasts with the avocado mixture and place the remaining cheese toasts on top, cheese-side up. Season with freshly ground black pepper and sprinkle with extra basil. Serve warm.

UNITS PER SERVE Grains **2** * Meat and alternatives **0** * Fruit **0** * Vegetables **0** * Dairy **2** * Fats and oils **1**

Swiss stuffed mushrooms on toast

Preparation: 15 minutes ✳ **Cooking:** 5 minutes
Difficulty: Easy

A

SERVES 4

12 medium-sized field mushrooms
   (about 75 g each)
light olive oil spray, for cooking
320 g Swiss cheese, coarsely grated
¼ cup chopped flat-leaf parsley
2 tablespoons thyme leaves
1 teaspoon freshly ground black pepper
8 x 40 g slices multigrain bread, toasted
2 tablespoons light margarine

Preheat the oven grill to high. Remove the stems from the mushrooms and finely chop, then tip into a bowl. Place the mushrooms, cup-side down, on a large non-stick baking tray and lightly spray with olive oil. Grill for 2 minutes. Remove the tray from the grill and carefully turn the mushrooms over so the cups are facing up.

Add the cheese, parsley, thyme and pepper to the bowl of chopped mushroom stems and stir to combine. Fill the mushroom cups with the cheese mixture and lightly spray with olive oil. Cook under the grill for 3 minutes or until the mushrooms are tender but not collapsing, and the cheese is melted and bubbling.

Evenly spread the toast with margarine and place on serving plates. Top with the stuffed mushrooms and serve warm.

UNITS PER SERVE Grains **2** ✳ Meat and alternatives **0** ✳ Fruit **0** ✳ Vegetables **1.5** ✳ Dairy **2** ✳ Fats and oils **1**

Hash with poached eggs

Preparation: 20 minutes ✳ **Cooking:** 20 minutes
Difficulty: Medium

B

SERVES 4

1 tablespoon olive oil
600 g orange sweet potato, peeled
    and cut into 1 cm pieces
1 onion, chopped
1 zucchini, chopped
340 g firm tofu, cut into 2 cm cubes
160 g haloumi, cut into 1 cm cubes
    (see Notes)
4 large eggs

CHIVE DRESSING
100 g low-fat natural Greek-style yoghurt
½ teaspoon Dijon mustard
¼ teaspoon ground turmeric (optional)
2 teaspoons white wine vinegar
2 tablespoons finely chopped chives

To make the chive dressing, place all the ingredients in a small bowl and whisk with a fork until smooth and well combined. Season with freshly ground black pepper and chill until you are ready to serve.

Heat half the olive oil in a large non-stick frying pan over medium–high heat. Add the sweet potato and cook, tossing occasionally, for 1 minute. Add 2 tablespoons water, cover and cook, shaking the pan occasionally, for 5 minutes or until the potato is just tender and the water has evaporated.

Add the onion, zucchini and tofu and cook, tossing occasionally, for 8 minutes or until the vegetables are tender and the tofu is golden. Add the haloumi and drizzle with the remaining olive oil. Cook, tossing occasionally, for 3–4 minutes or until the haloumi has softened and is nicely golden.

Meanwhile, bring a deep frying pan of water to a very gentle simmer. Individually crack each egg into a small cup or bowl, gently slide into the water and poach for 1 minute or until the whites have set but the yolk is still runny. Transfer the eggs to a plate with a slotted spoon.

Divide the vegetable hash among serving plates, top with the poached eggs and drizzle with the chive dressing. Serve warm.

NOTES

This chive dressing is a great alternative to the hollandaise sauce usually served with poached eggs, and can be made up to 2 days ahead. Keep chilled in an airtight container and stir well before serving.

If preferred, you can omit the tofu and replace it with an additional poached egg (2 eggs per person).

If you want to reduce the salt content of the haloumi, place the cubes in a bowl of water for 30 minutes to steep. Drain before use.

UNITS PER SERVE Grains **1** ✳ Meat and alternatives **1** ✳ Fruit **0** ✳ Vegetables **0.5** ✳ Dairy **1** ✳ Fats and oils **1**

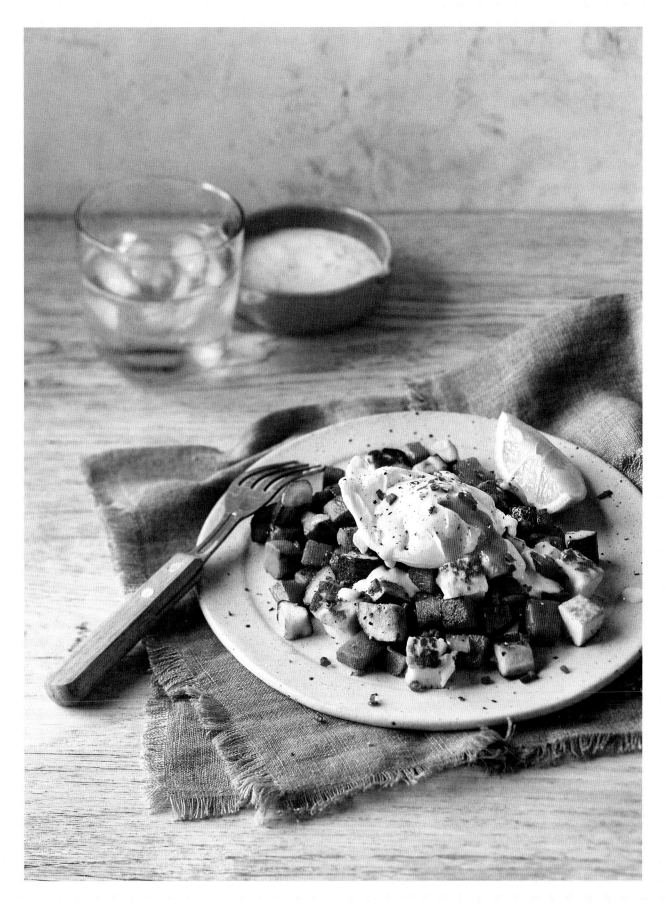

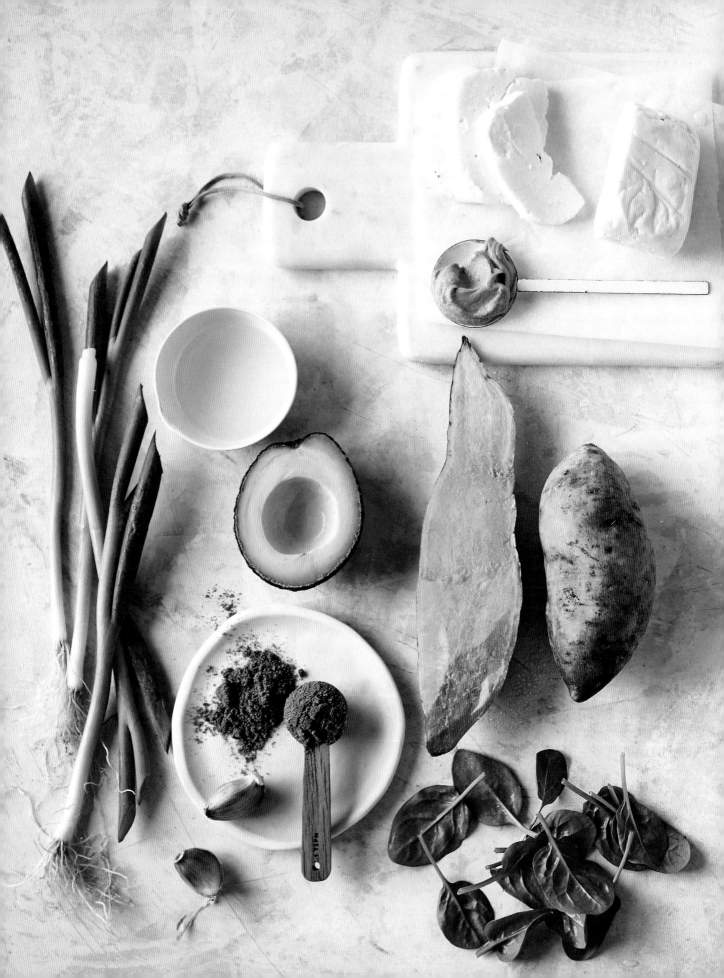

Sweet potato and haloumi fritters

Preparation: 15 minutes * **Cooking:** 25 minutes
Difficulty: Medium

— A —

SERVES 4

1.2 kg orange sweet potato, peeled and coarsely grated
320 g haloumi, coarsely grated (see Notes)
2 teaspoons ground cumin
light olive oil spray, for cooking
2 cloves garlic, crushed
4 spring onions, white part thinly sliced into rounds, green part thinly sliced diagonally
120 g baby spinach leaves

AVOCADO DRESSING

½ (80 g) medium-sized avocado
⅓ cup (80 ml) white wine vinegar or apple cider vinegar
½ teaspoon Dijon mustard

UNITS PER SERVE

Grains 2 * Meat and alternatives 0
Fruit 0 * Vegetables 0.5
Dairy 2 * Fats and oils 1

To make the avocado dressing, blend all the ingredients in a jug with a hand-held blender until smooth. Season with black pepper and set aside.

Heat a large non-stick frying pan over low–medium heat. Combine the sweet potato, haloumi and cumin in a bowl and season with freshly ground black pepper. Lightly spray the pan with olive oil and drop in firmly packed ½ cup measures of the sweet potato mixture, pressing down to form 8 cm circles. Depending on the size of your pan, you will probably need to do this in two batches of four. Cook for 5 minutes each side or until golden and cooked through. Remove and cover to keep warm.

Lightly spray the pan with a little more oil and increase the heat to high. Add the garlic, white part of the spring onion, spinach and ¼ cup (60 ml) water. Cook, tossing constantly, for 2 minutes or until the spinach has just wilted. Remove the pan from the heat and season with black pepper.

Serve two sweet potato fritters per person, layered with the spinach mixture. Spoon over the dressing and sprinkle with the green spring onion.

NOTES

If you want to reduce the salt content of the haloumi, place the block in a bowl of water for 30 minutes to steep. Drain before use.

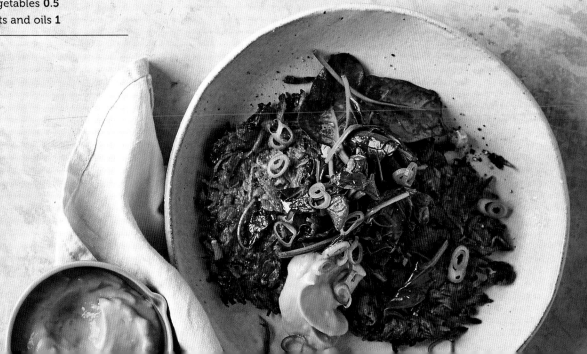

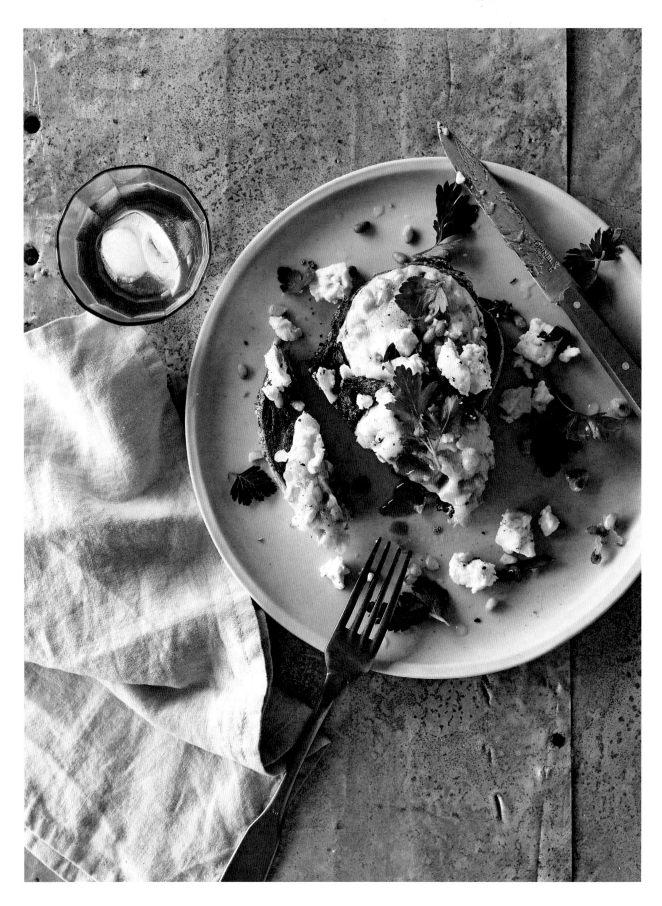

Corn fritters with feta

Preparation: 20 minutes * **Cooking:** 10 minutes
Difficulty: Medium

B

SERVES 4

160 g reduced-fat feta,
    cut into 1 cm pieces (see Notes)
2 tablespoons red wine vinegar
1 cup flat-leaf parsley leaves
28 g pine nuts, toasted
olive oil spray, for cooking
8 large eggs
2 cobs sweetcorn, husks and silks
    removed, kernels sliced off
80 g tasty cheese, grated
4 x 40 g slices multigrain bread, toasted

Combine the feta, vinegar, parsley and pine nuts in a bowl and season with freshly ground black pepper. Set aside.

Lightly spray a large non-stick frying pan with olive oil and place over medium heat. Liberally spray four 7 cm egg rings with oil and place in the pan. You'll be cooking the fritters in two batches.

Crack an egg into each egg ring, then top with some of the corn kernels and cheese. Cook for 2 minutes, then flip and cook for a further 1 minute or until the whites have set, the yolks are still a little runny, and the cheese is melted and golden. Carefully remove the fritters from the rings, place on a plate and cover to keep warm. Spray the egg rings again and repeat with the remaining eggs, corn and cheese to make eight fritters in total.

Divide the fritters among serving plates and spoon over the feta mixture. Serve warm with toast.

NOTES

If you want to reduce the salt content of the feta, cut it into cubes and place in a bowl of water for 30 minutes to steep. Drain before use.

UNITS PER SERVE Grains **1** * Meat and alternatives **1** * Fruit **0** * Vegetables **1** * Dairy **1** * Fats and oils **1**

Tortilla with salsa

Preparation: 20 minutes, plus resting time ✳ **Cooking:** 35 minutes
Difficulty: Medium

B

SERVES 4

600 g baby potatoes
1 tablespoon olive oil
1 red onion, chopped
8 large eggs
½ cup (125 ml) evaporated skim milk
80 g cheddar, crumbled
200 g low-fat natural Greek-style yoghurt
basil leaves, to serve (optional)

SALSA
2 spring onions, white and green
    parts thinly sliced
250 g cherry tomatoes, quartered
2 tablespoons red wine vinegar
½ cup basil leaves

To make the salsa, combine all the ingredients in a bowl. Season with freshly ground black pepper and set aside.

Cook the potatoes in a large saucepan of boiling water for 12–15 minutes or until just tender. Drain and cool slightly before cutting in half.

Heat the olive oil in a 22 cm flameproof non-stick frying pan over medium heat. Add the onion and cook, stirring occasionally, for 3 minutes or until starting to soften. Add the potato and cook, tossing occasionally, for 5 minutes or until golden and crisp.

While the potato is cooking, whisk together the eggs and milk in a jug. Season with freshly ground black pepper.

Reduce the heat to low. Pour the egg mixture over the potato and onion and cook, gently stirring occasionally, for 1 minute. Sprinkle over the cheddar and cook, untouched, for 8–10 minutes or until the egg has set firmly in the centre.

Meanwhile, preheat the oven grill to high.

Transfer the pan to the grill and cook for a further 2 minutes or until the top is set and golden. Remove and leave to rest for 5 minutes before turning out and slicing.

Serve the tortilla warm topped with yoghurt, salsa and a sprinkling of basil leaves, if desired.

NOTES

You can cook the potatoes up to 1 day ahead. Simply cool and keep chilled in an airtight container until you are ready to make the tortilla.

UNITS PER SERVE Grains **1** ✳ Meat and alternatives **1** ✳ Fruit **0** ✳ Vegetables **1.5** ✳ Dairy **1** ✳ Fats and oils **1**

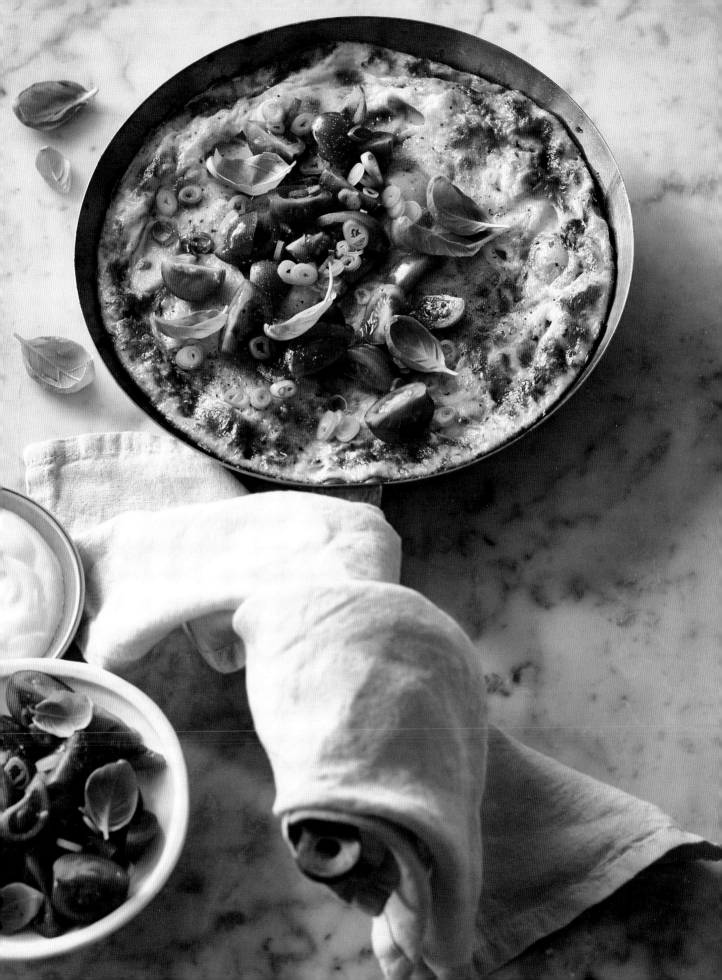

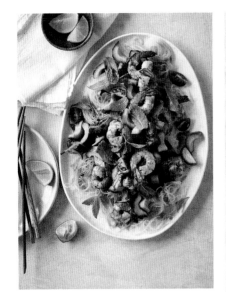

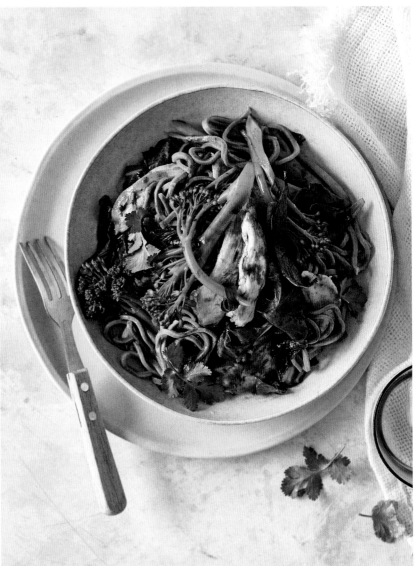

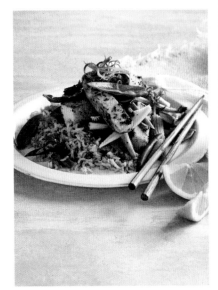

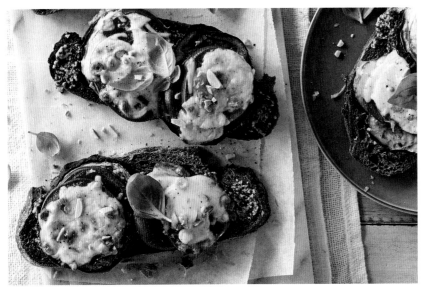

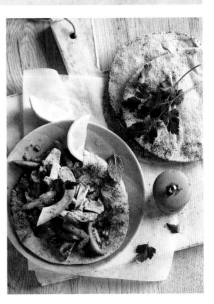

2. Lunch

Polenta-crumbed fish lettuce wraps

Preparation: 25 minutes, plus chilling time ✴ **Cooking:** 10 minutes
Difficulty: Medium

A

SERVES 4

1 large egg
¼ cup (40 g) fine instant polenta
½ cup chopped dill
400 g firm white fish fillets, skin removed
    and pin-boned, cut into 2 cm pieces
1 tablespoon light margarine
2 teaspoons olive oil
70 g large wholemeal wraps, halved
4 butter lettuce leaves
300 g cherry tomatoes,
    halved or quartered
2 cups (100 g) mixed salad sprouts
lime wedges, to serve

MUSTARD DRESSING
4 spring onions, white and
    green parts thinly sliced
2 teaspoons wholegrain mustard
⅓ cup (80 ml) white wine vinegar

To make the mustard dressing, combine all the ingredients in a small jug. Season with freshly ground black pepper and set aside.

Using a fork, whisk the egg and 1 tablespoon water in a shallow dish. Season with freshly ground black pepper. Combine the polenta and dill in a separate shallow dish and season with freshly ground black pepper.

Working in batches, dip the fish in the egg mixture, turning to coat well, then transfer to the polenta mixture to lightly coat on all sides, pressing down firmly to help it adhere. Transfer to a plate, then cover and chill for 20 minutes to set the crumb.

Heat the margarine and oil in a large non-stick frying pan over medium heat. Add the fish and cook, turning occasionally, for 8–10 minutes or until just cooked and golden. Transfer to a heatproof plate.

Divide the wrap halves among serving plates, then top with lettuce leaves, tomatoes, sprouts and the warm fish. Spoon over the mustard dressing and serve with lime wedges alongside.

UNITS PER SERVE Grains **1** ✴ Meat and alternatives **1** ✴ Fruit **0** ✴ Vegetables **2** ✴ Dairy **0** ✴ Fats and oils **1**

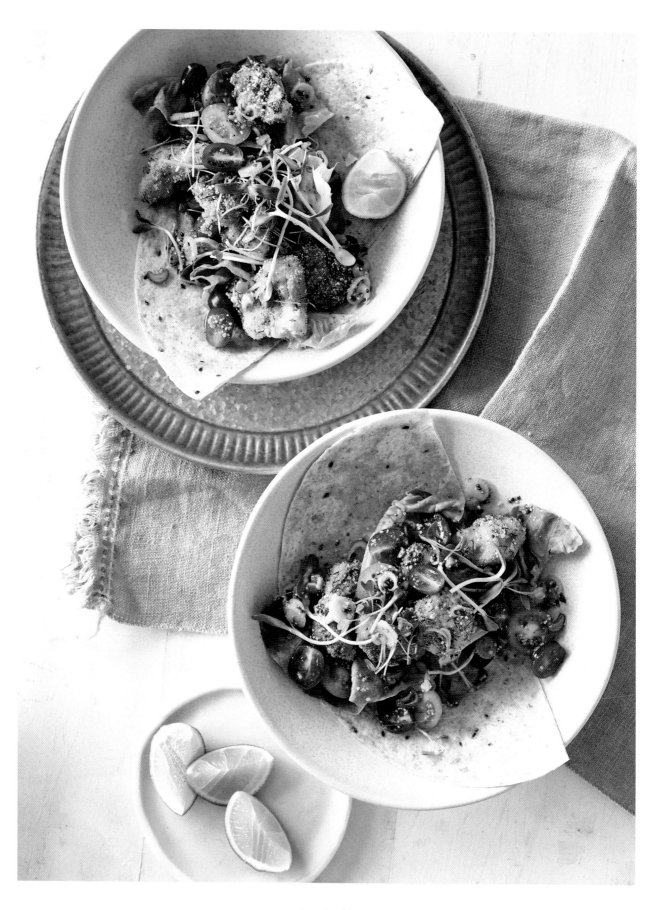

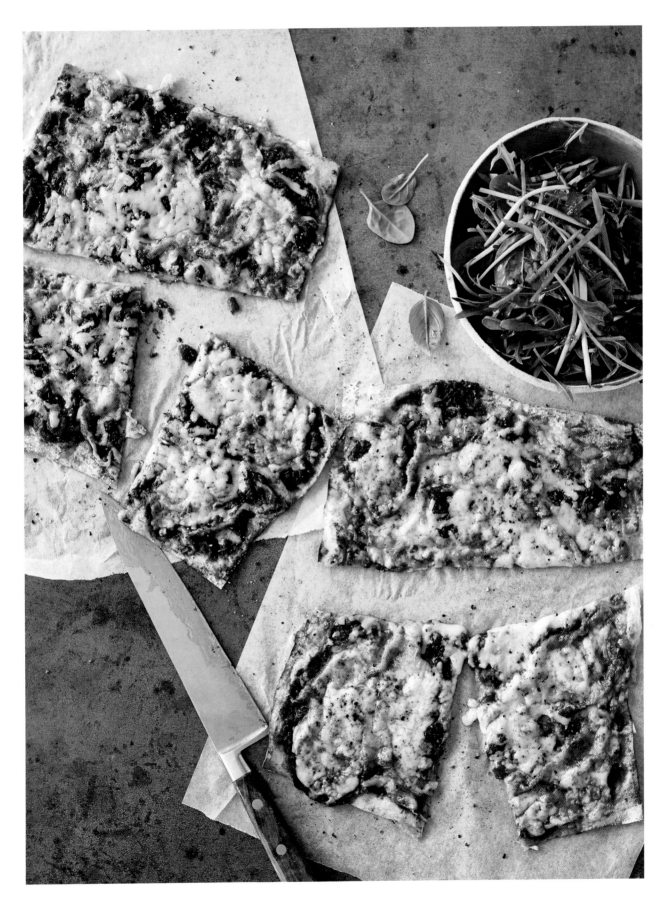

Mountain bread pizzas

Preparation: 20 minutes ✳ **Cooking:** 20 minutes
Difficulty: Easy

B

SERVES 4

1 tablespoon extra virgin olive oil
2 teaspoons balsamic vinegar
1 small clove garlic, crushed
¼ teaspoon dried chilli flakes (optional)
2 zucchini, peeled into long thin ribbons
8 x 25 g wholemeal or rye
    mountain breads
320 g tasty cheese, coarsely grated
1 x 400 g tin chopped tomatoes
    with basil and garlic
1 carrot, peeled into long thin ribbons
1½ cups (45 g) baby spinach and rocket
    salad leaf mix

Preheat the oven to 180°C (160°C fan-forced). Line two large baking trays with baking paper.

Using a fork, whisk together the olive oil, vinegar, garlic and chilli flakes (if using) in a large bowl. Add the zucchini and season with freshly ground black pepper. Toss to combine, then set aside, tossing occasionally.

Lay two mountain breads side by side on each tray and sprinkle evenly with half the cheese. Place the remaining breads on top to cover. Spoon over the chopped tomato and sprinkle with the remaining cheese. Bake for 15–20 minutes or until the breads are crisp and the cheese is melted, bubbling and golden.

Add the carrot and salad leaves to the zucchini mixture and toss to combine. Serve alongside the pizzas.

UNITS PER SERVE Grains **2** ✳ Meat and alternatives **0** ✳ Fruit **0** ✳ Vegetables **3.5** ✳ Dairy **2** ✳ Fats and oils **1**

PORTABLE SALADS

— A —

All recipes serve 1.
Prep, then layer the ingredients in a portable airtight
glass jar with a lid, and store in the fridge overnight.
To serve, tip the salad into a bowl and toss to combine.
A convenient way to prepare a nutritious lunch in advance!

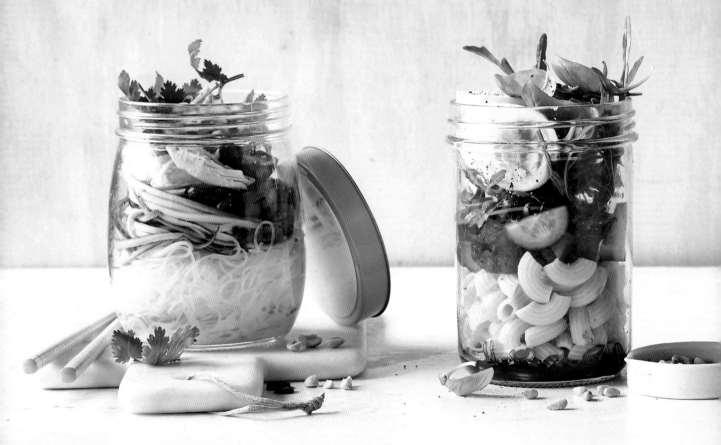

Chicken noodle salad

Layer in order the finely grated zest and juice of 1 large
lemon; ¼ teaspoon sesame oil; 30 g rice vermicelli,
soaked, broken into 5 cm lengths; 1 small zucchini,
coarsely grated; 1 tomato, chopped; 100 g cooked
chicken breast fillet, sliced; 1 long red chilli, seeded and
chopped; 1 teaspoon grated ginger; ¼ cup coriander
leaves and 7 g finely chopped toasted peanuts.

UNITS PER SERVE

Grains **1** ✱ Meat and alternatives **1** ✱ Fruit **0**
Vegetables **3** ✱ Dairy **0** ✱ Fats and oils **1**

Egg and pasta salad

Layer in order ¼ cup (60 ml) balsamic vinegar;
½ cup (80 g) cooked small elbow macaroni;
1 small Lebanese cucumber, sliced; ¼ small red
onion, thinly sliced; ½ cup (15 g) baby rocket leaves;
2 large hard-boiled eggs, halved; ⅓ cup small basil
leaves and 7 g toasted pine nuts.

UNITS PER SERVE

Grains **1** ✱ Meat and alternatives **1** ✱ Fruit **0**
Vegetables **3** ✱ Dairy **0** ✱ Fats and oils **1**

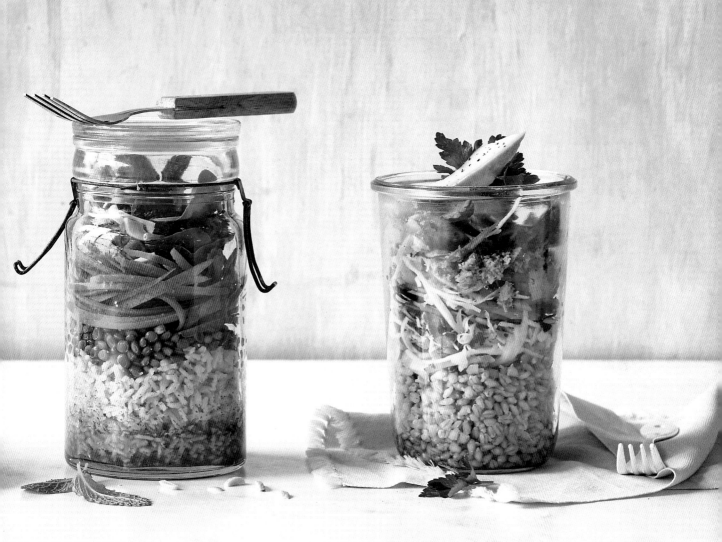

Lentil and rice salad

Layer in order 1 teaspoon korma curry paste; ¼ cup (60 ml) white wine vinegar; ½ cup (100 g) cooked brown basmati rice; 150 g drained, rinsed tinned lentils; 1 small carrot, grated; 2 spring onions, thinly sliced; 1 cup (30 g) baby spinach leaves; 2 tablespoons chopped mint and 7 g toasted slivered almonds.

UNITS PER SERVE

Grains **1** ✽ Meat and alternatives **1** ✽ Fruit **0**
Vegetables **2** ✽ Dairy **0** ✽ Fats and oils **1**

Tuna barley slaw

Layer in order ¼ cup (60 ml) red wine vinegar; ½ cup (60 g) cooked barley; 1 cup (100 g) fresh coleslaw salad mix; 1 stick celery, thinly sliced; 100 g drained tuna chunks in spring water; ½ cup flat-leaf parsley leaves and 20 g sliced avocado.

UNITS PER SERVE

Grains **1** ✽ Meat and alternatives **1** ✽ Fruit **0**
Vegetables **2.5** ✽ Dairy **0** ✽ Fats and oils **1**

Tuna caponata crispbreads

Preparation: 20 minutes ✳ **Cooking:** 15 minutes
Difficulty: Easy

A

SERVES 4

1 tablespoon olive oil
1 clove garlic, crushed
1 eggplant, chopped
1 small red capsicum, seeded
   and chopped
1 red onion, chopped
2 sticks celery, chopped
2 teaspoons salt-reduced tomato paste
¼ cup (60 ml) red wine vinegar
2 tablespoons baby capers in brine,
   rinsed and chopped
1 x 400 g tin tuna chunks in springwater,
   drained and thickly flaked
½ cup flat-leaf parsley leaves
12 high-fibre crispbreads, such as Ryvita
lemon wedges, to serve

Heat the olive oil in a large non-stick frying pan over medium–high heat. Add the garlic, eggplant, capsicum, onion and celery and cook, stirring occasionally, for 10 minutes or until softened and golden.

Add the tomato paste and cook, stirring, for 30 seconds. Remove the pan from the heat and immediately stir in the vinegar until well combined.

Add the capers, tuna and parsley and stir gently to combine. Season with freshly ground black pepper. Spoon evenly over the crispbreads and serve with lemon wedges alongside.

UNITS PER SERVE Grains **1** ✳ Meat and alternatives **1** ✳ Fruit **0** ✳ Vegetables **3.5** ✳ Dairy **0** ✳ Fats and oils **1**

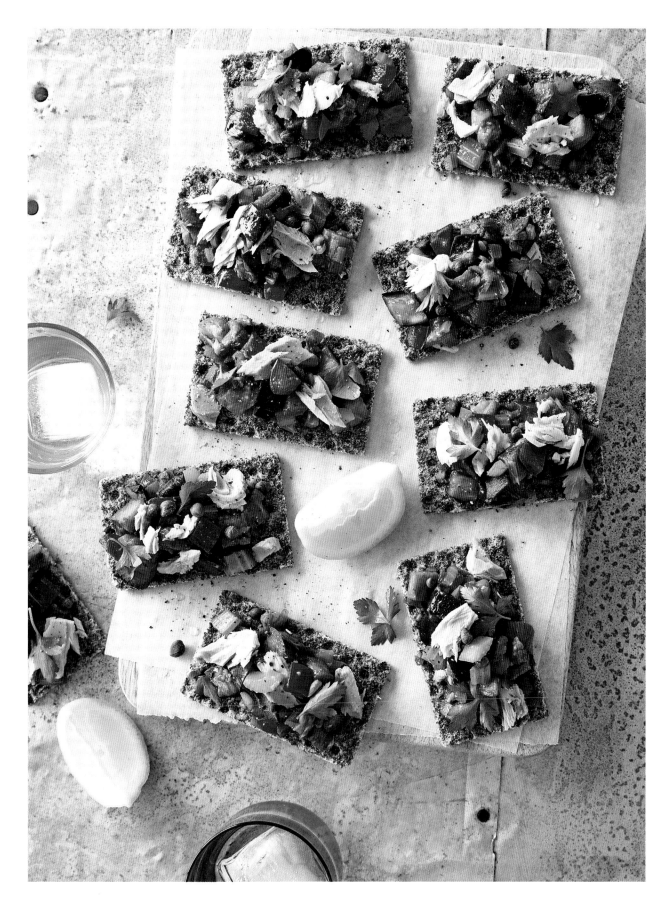

Beef and barley salad with pickled beetroot beans

Preparation: 20 minutes, plus resting time ✳ **Cooking:** 35 minutes
Difficulty: Easy

A

⅔ cup (120 g) pearl barley

1 tablespoon extra virgin olive oil

¼ cup (60 ml) white wine vinegar

1 teaspoon Dijon mustard

1 x 450 g tin diced beetroot, drained

300 g drained tinned cannellini beans
(see Notes)

200 g lean beef fillet steak

light olive oil spray, for cooking

2 teaspoons freshly ground black pepper

4 spring onions, white and green parts
thinly sliced

2 cups (60 g) baby spinach and
rocket salad mix

Cook the barley in a large saucepan of boiling water for 20–25 minutes or until tender. Drain, then rinse well under cold running water. Drain again, then place in a large bowl and set aside.

Meanwhile, using a fork, whisk together the olive oil, vinegar and mustard in a bowl. Add the beetroot and cannellini beans and toss well to combine. Season with freshly ground black pepper, then set aside for 20 minutes to marinate.

Preheat a chargrill pan over high heat. Lightly spray both sides of the steak with oil, then coat in the pepper. Chargrill for 3 minutes each side for medium or until cooked to your liking. Transfer to a plate and leave to rest, covered, for 5 minutes. Cut the steak in half, then very thinly slice crossways into strips. Add the steak to the barley in the bowl, along with any resting juices on the plate.

Add the spring onion and salad mix to the barley mixture and toss well to combine. Divide among serving bowls and spoon the beetroot mixture alongside.

NOTES

You will need two 400 g tins of cannellini beans for this recipe. Store any leftover beans in an airtight container in the fridge for up to 3 days or in an airtight container in the freezer for up to 3 months.

UNITS PER SERVE Grains **1** ✳ Meat and alternatives **1** ✳ Fruit **0** ✳ Vegetables **2** ✳ Dairy **0** ✳ Fats and oils **1**

Parmesan polenta with grilled mushrooms

Preparation: 15 minutes * **Cooking:** 10 minutes
Difficulty: Medium

B

SERVES 4

800 g mixed mushrooms (field, button,
   Swiss brown), wiped clean and halved
2 tablespoons thyme leaves
2 cloves garlic, thinly sliced
light olive oil spray, for cooking
1 litre low-fat milk
1 cup (170 g) fine (instant) polenta
2 tablespoons light margarine
160 g parmesan, coarsely grated
2 sourdough bread rolls, halved
   horizontally and toasted
2 cups (60 g) baby rocket leaves

Preheat the oven grill to high. Place the mushrooms on a large non-stick baking tray and sprinkle with the thyme and garlic. Lightly spray with olive oil and season with freshly ground black pepper. Cook under the grill, turning once, for 8–10 minutes or until tender and light golden.

Meanwhile, combine the milk and 2 cups (500 ml) water in a large saucepan over medium–high heat. Bring to the boil, then immediately pour in the polenta while whisking constantly. Cook, whisking vigorously, for 2–3 minutes or until the mixture has thickened.

Remove the pan from the heat and add the margarine and three-quarters of the parmesan. Use a wooden spoon to vigorously stir for 1 minute or until melted and combined.

Divide the polenta among serving bowls and spoon over the mushroom mixture and any pan juices. Top with the remaining parmesan and serve with the toasted rolls and rocket leaves.

UNITS PER SERVE Grains **2** * Meat and alternatives **0** * Fruit **0** * Vegetables **2** * Dairy **2** * Fats and oils **1**

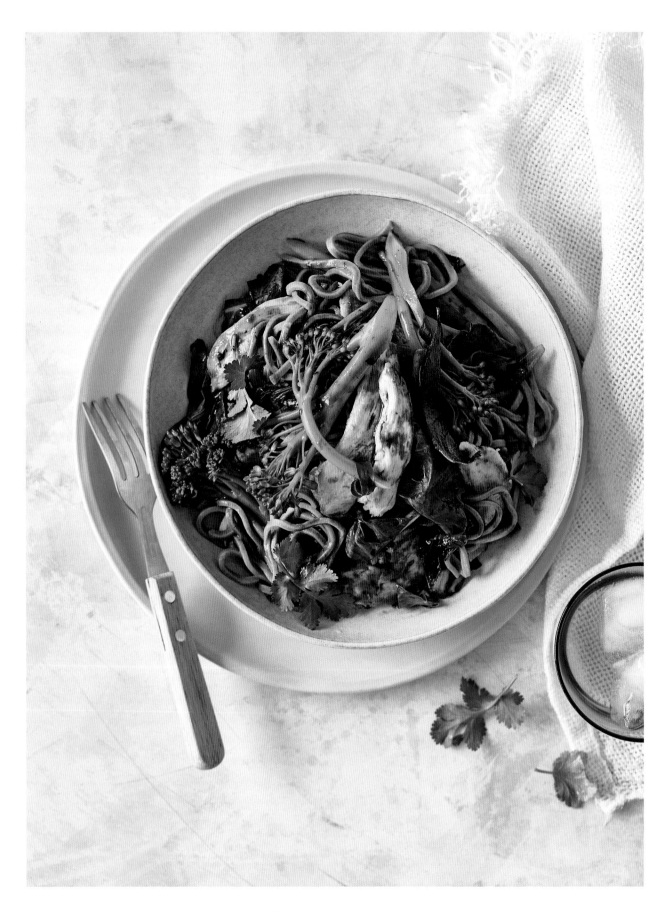

Chicken soba noodles

Preparation: 15 minutes ✻ **Cooking:** 10 minutes
Difficulty: Easy

A

3 teaspoons sunflower oil

1 teaspoon sesame oil

400 g lean chicken breast fillet,
    thinly sliced crossways

1 red onion, cut into wedges

1 bunch Chinese broccoli, trimmed,
    stems thinly sliced and leaves torn

2 tablespoons salt-reduced hoisin sauce

1 tablespoon salt-reduced soy sauce

2 teaspoons finely grated ginger

1 x 180 g packet shelf-fresh soba noodles

1 bunch broccolini, trimmed,
    stalks halved lengthways, then
    halved crossways

½ cup small coriander sprigs

Heat the sunflower and sesame oils in a large wok over high heat. Add the chicken and stir-fry for 3–4 minutes. Add the onion and cook for 1 minute.

Add the Chinese broccoli, hoisin, soy sauce, ginger and 2 tablespoons water. Stir-fry for 2 minutes or until the chicken is cooked and the vegetables are just tender.

Meanwhile, bring a large saucepan of water to the boil over high heat. Add the noodles and broccolini and cook for 1–2 minutes or until the noodles are heated through and separate easily, and the broccoli is just tender. Drain well, then divide among serving bowls.

Spoon the chicken mixture over the noodles, top with coriander and serve.

UNITS PER SERVE Grains **1** ✻ Meat and alternatives **1** ✻ Fruit **0** ✻ Vegetables **2** ✻ Dairy **0** ✻ Fats and oils **1**

Lamb and silverbeet risoni

Preparation: 20 minutes, plus resting time ✳ **Cooking:** 20 minutes
Difficulty: Easy

A

SERVES 4

⅔ cup (130 g) risoni
2 tablespoons chopped flat-leaf parsley
2 tablespoons chopped mint
light olive oil spray, for cooking
400 g lamb backstrap
3 teaspoons Moroccan spice seasoning
1 bunch asparagus, trimmed
1 tablespoon olive oil
1 leek, white part only, thinly
    sliced into rounds
2 teaspoons salt-reduced tomato paste
1 bunch silverbeet, trimmed, white cores
    removed and leaves torn
2 tablespoons red wine vinegar

Cook the risoni in a large saucepan of boiling water over high heat for 6–8 minutes or until just tender. Drain, then cool under cold running water. Drain well and transfer to a large heatproof bowl. Stir in the parsley and mint and season with freshly ground black pepper.

Meanwhile, preheat a large non-stick frying pan over medium–high heat.

Lightly spray the olive oil over both sides of the lamb, then sprinkle with 2 teaspoons of the spice seasoning. Add the lamb and asparagus to the pan and cook, turning once, for 5 minutes or until the asparagus is just tender and the lamb is cooked to medium. Transfer the lamb and asparagus to a heatproof plate, cover loosely with foil and leave to rest for 5 minutes, then thinly slice the lamb. Add the asparagus, lamb and any resting juices to the risoni mixture in the bowl. Toss well to combine.

Heat the tablespoon of olive oil in the same pan. Add the leek and cook, stirring occasionally, for 2 minutes or until starting to soften. Stir in the tomato paste and remaining spice seasoning and cook for 1 minute or until fragrant. Add the silverbeet and 2 tablespoons water and cook, tossing, for 1–2 minutes or until the silverbeet is just wilted. Remove the pan from the heat and stir through the vinegar.

Divide everything among four serving bowls and serve warm.

UNITS PER SERVE Grains **1** ✳ Meat and alternatives **1** ✳ Fruit **0** ✳ Vegetables **2** ✳ Dairy **0** ✳ Fats and oils **1**

Lemon and broccolini cheesy rice

Preparation: 10 minutes, plus cooling time ✳ **Cooking:** 30 minutes
Difficulty: Medium

B

1 tablespoon light margarine
2 teaspoons olive oil
1 large leek, trimmed, white and green
   parts thinly sliced into rounds
2 cloves garlic, crushed
1½ cups (320 g) arborio rice
4 cups (1 litre) low-fat milk
about 3 cups (750 ml) salt-reduced
   vegetable stock, heated
2 bunches broccolini, trimmed
   and cut into 4 cm lengths
finely grated zest and juice of
   1 large lemon
120 g cheddar, crumbled
40 g parmesan, finely grated
¼ cup small flat-leaf parsley leaves

Heat the margarine and olive oil in a large heavy-based saucepan over low–medium heat. Add the leek and garlic and cook, stirring occasionally, for 10 minutes or until softened and light golden. Add the rice and stir for 1 minute or until the rice grains are well coated in the oil mixture.

Reduce the heat to low. Gradually add the milk, ½ cup (125 ml) at a time, stirring constantly until it has been completely absorbed before adding the next batch. Then add the hot stock ½ cup (125 ml) at a time, stirring constantly until it has been completely absorbed before adding the next batch. When you are about halfway through the stock, add the broccolini. Continue adding the stock in batches and cook until the rice is just tender, about 15–18 minutes all up. (Depending on your rice, you may need to use all of the stock, or you may find there is some left over.) As soon as the rice is tender, remove the pan from the heat and immediately add the lemon zest and juice, cheddar and parmesan, stirring until the cheeses melt.

Divide the cheesy rice among large serving bowls. Season with freshly ground black pepper and serve sprinkled with parsley.

UNITS PER SERVE Grains **2** ✳ Meat and alternatives **0** ✳ Fruit **0** ✳ Vegetables **2** ✳ Dairy **2** ✳ Fats and oils **1**

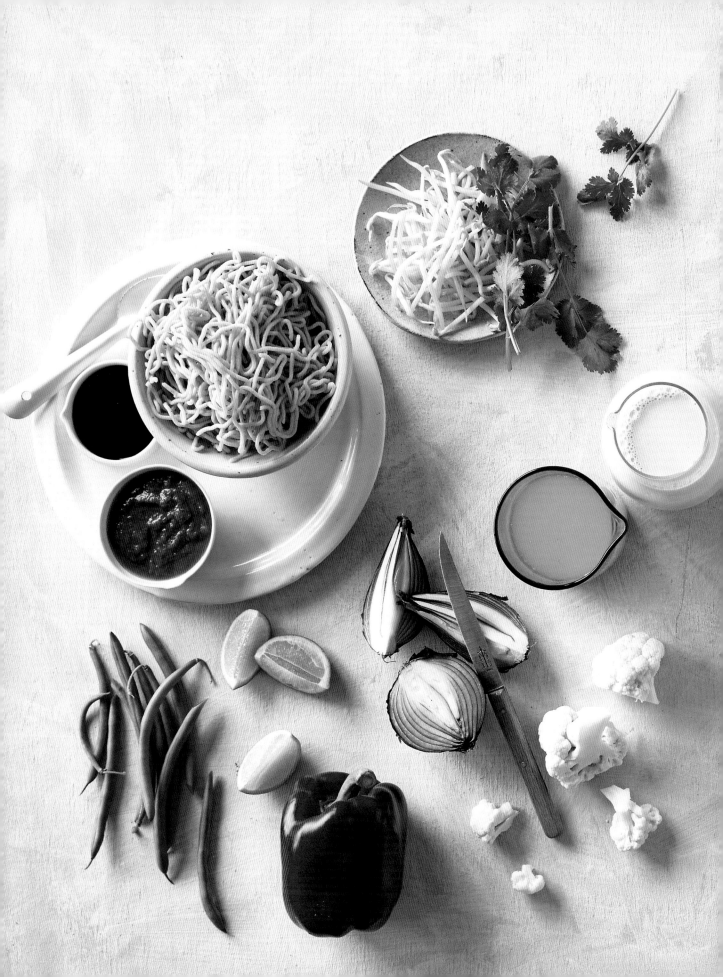

Quick veggie laksa

Preparation: 15 minutes ✱ **Cooking:** 10 minutes
Difficulty: Easy

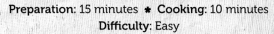

SERVES 4

¼ cup (75 g) Thai-style
    laksa curry paste
1 red onion, cut into thin wedges
1 cup (100 g) small cauliflower florets
    (about ¼ head cauliflower)
960 ml light and creamy coconut
    evaporated milk (see Notes)
2 cups (500 ml) salt-reduced
    vegetable stock
2 tablespoons salt-reduced soy sauce
1 small red capsicum, seeded
    and chopped
400 g shelf-fresh wholegrain noodles
200 g baby green beans, trimmed
1 cup (80 g) bean sprouts, trimmed
1 cup small coriander sprigs
lime wedges, to serve

UNITS PER SERVE

Grains 2 ✱ Meat and alternatives 0
Fruit 0 ✱ Vegetables 2 ✱ Dairy 2
Fats and oils 1

Heat the curry paste in a large saucepan over medium–high heat. Add the onion and cook, stirring, for 1 minute or until fragrant. Add the cauliflower, evaporated milk and stock. Reduce the heat to low–medium and simmer gently for 5 minutes or until the cauliflower is just tender. Stir in the soy sauce and capsicum, then remove the pan from the heat.

Meanwhile, cook the noodles and green beans in a large saucepan of boiling water for 2–3 minutes or until the noodles are heated through and separate easily, and the beans are just tender. Drain well, then divide among large serving bowls.

Add the bean sprouts to the bowls and ladle over the cauliflower mixture. Top with coriander and serve with lime wedges.

NOTES

You will need three 375 ml tins of coconut evaporated milk for this recipe. Store the leftover milk in an airtight container in the fridge for up to 1 week.

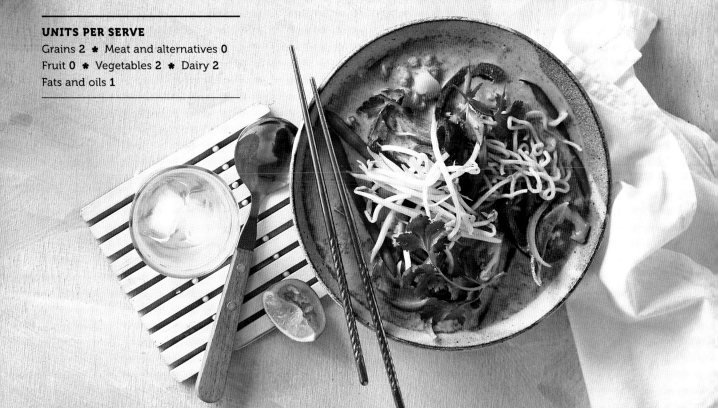

Capsicum and feta-stuffed rolls

Preparation: 20 minutes, plus cooling and overnight chilling time ✳ **Cooking:** 10 minutes
Difficulty: Medium

B

SERVES 4

1 tablespoon olive oil

1 clove garlic, crushed

2 spring onions, white and green
parts thinly sliced

1 small red capsicum, seeded
and cut into 1 cm thick strips

1 small green capsicum, seeded
and cut into 1 cm thick strips

2 tablespoons chopped rosemary

¼ cup (60 ml) white wine vinegar

4 medium-sized crusty round
multigrain rolls

160 g cheddar, crumbled

320 g reduced-fat feta, crumbled
(see Notes)

1½ cups (45 g) mixed salad leaves

2 Lebanese cucumbers, cut into long
thin ribbons using a vegetable peeler

lemon wedges, to serve

Heat the olive oil in a medium saucepan over medium–high heat. Add the garlic, spring onion and red and green capsicum and cook, stirring occasionally, for 5–8 minutes or until softened and light golden. Transfer to a heatproof bowl and add the rosemary and vinegar. Season with freshly ground black pepper and stir until well combined, then set aside to cool.

With the rolls sitting flat on a board, use a serrated knife to cut their tops off, by about 1.5 cm. Using your fingers, remove the soft insides and pull apart into large crumbs. Add the fresh crumbs to the capsicum mixture, then add the cheddar and feta and stir until well combined.

Spoon the capsicum mixture into the roll shells, packing it down firmly. Replace the lids, then tightly wrap each filled roll in plastic film. Place the rolls on a small baking tray, rest another baking tray on top and weigh it down with two or three food tins (such as tomatoes or beans). Place in the fridge and chill for a few hours or overnight if you have time.

Toss together the mixed leaves and cucumber. Cut the stuffed rolls in half and serve with the salad and lemon wedges.

NOTES

You can make a double batch of this recipe and keep the rolls individually wrapped in an airtight container in the fridge for up to 3 days.

If you want to reduce the salt content of the feta, cut it into cubes and place in a bowl of water for 30 minutes to steep. Drain before use.

UNITS PER SERVE Grains **2** ✳ Meat and alternatives **0** ✳ Fruit **0** ✳ Vegetables **2.5** ✳ Dairy **2** ✳ Fats and oils **1**

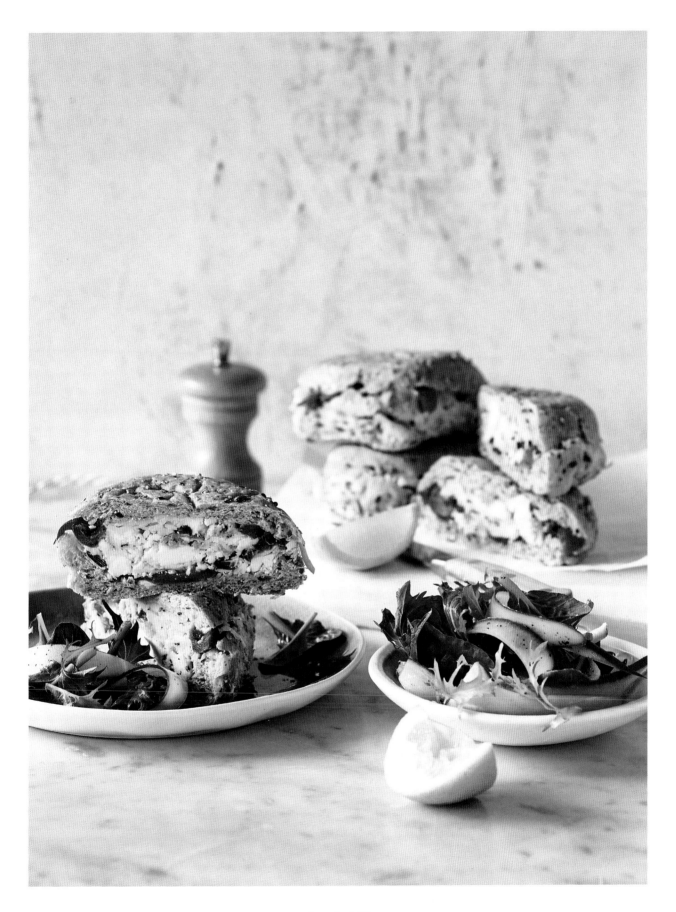

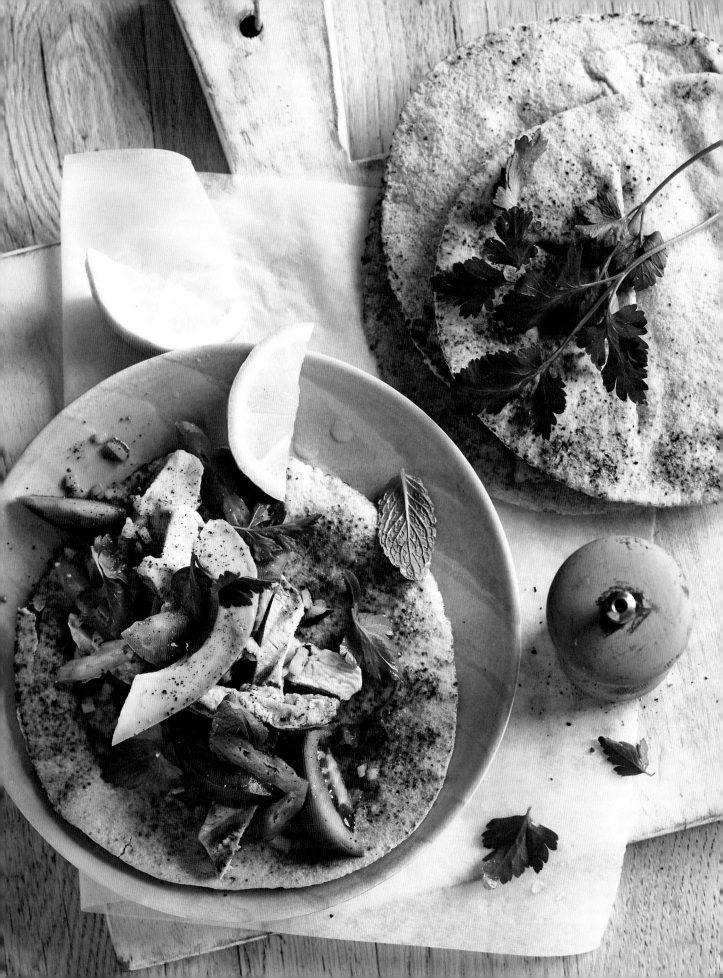

Chicken and parsley salad pitas

Preparation: 15 minutes, plus resting time ✳ **Cooking:** 10 minutes
Difficulty: Easy

A

SERVES 4

¼ cup (60 ml) white wine vinegar
1 small red onion, finely chopped
1 teaspoon Dijon mustard
1 teaspoon harissa spice seasoning
400 g lean chicken breast fillet,
    halved horizontally
2 sticks celery, thinly sliced
1 cup small flat-leaf parsley leaves
½ cup small mint leaves
2 ripe tomatoes, chopped
4 x 40 g wholemeal pita breads
80 g avocado, chopped

Using a fork, whisk together the vinegar, onion, mustard and harissa seasoning in a large heatproof bowl. Set aside.

Preheat a chargrill pan over medium–high heat. Add the chicken and cook, turning once, for 8 minutes or until golden and cooked through. Transfer to a plate, cover loosely with foil and rest for 5 minutes. Thinly slice, then add to the onion mixture in the bowl, along with any resting juices on the plate.

Add the celery, parsley, mint and tomato to the chicken mixture and gently toss to combine. Spoon evenly onto the pita bread, top with the avocado and serve.

UNITS PER SERVE Grains **1** ✳ Meat and alternatives **1** ✳ Fruit **0** ✳ Vegetables **2** ✳ Dairy **0** ✳ Fats and oils **1**

Eggplant parmigiana toasts

Preparation: 15 minutes　✻　**Cooking:** 30 minutes
Difficulty: Easy

B

SERVES 4

2 eggplants, sliced into rounds

light olive oil spray, for cooking

4 tomatoes, thinly sliced into rounds

2 spring onions, white and green
 parts thinly sliced

320 g firm mozzarella, coarsely grated

8 x 40 g slices crunchy wholemeal
 sourdough, toasted

2 tablespoons wholegrain mustard

28 g slivered almonds, toasted and
 roughly chopped

1 teaspoon finely grated lemon zest

1 cup basil leaves

Preheat the oven grill to high. Lightly spray the eggplant slices on both sides with olive oil and arrange in a single layer on two large non-stick baking trays. Grill each tray, turning the slices once, for 8–10 minutes or until cooked and golden. Remove and season with freshly ground black pepper.

Place two tomato slices on top of each eggplant slice and grill each tray for a further 1 minute. Top with spring onion and season with freshly ground black pepper, then sprinkle over the mozzarella. Grill each tray for 2–3 minutes or until the cheese is melted and bubbling.

Divide the toast among four serving plates and spread evenly with the mustard. Top with the hot eggplant slices, then sprinkle with the almonds and lemon zest. Serve warm, scattered with basil leaves.

UNITS PER SERVE Grains **2** ✻ Meat and alternatives **0** ✻ Fruit **0** ✻ Vegetables **4** ✻ Dairy **2** ✻ Fats and oils **1**

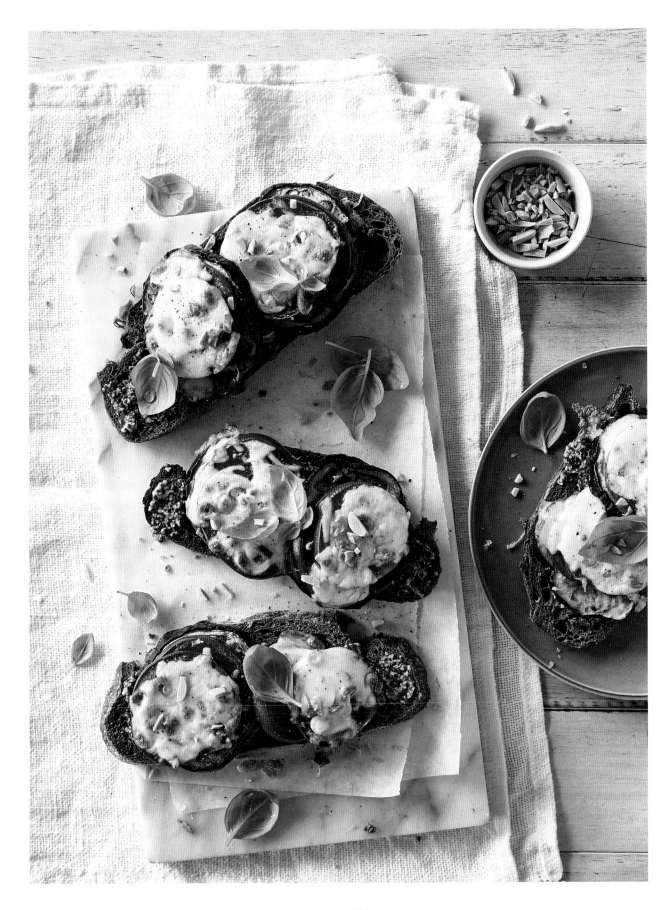

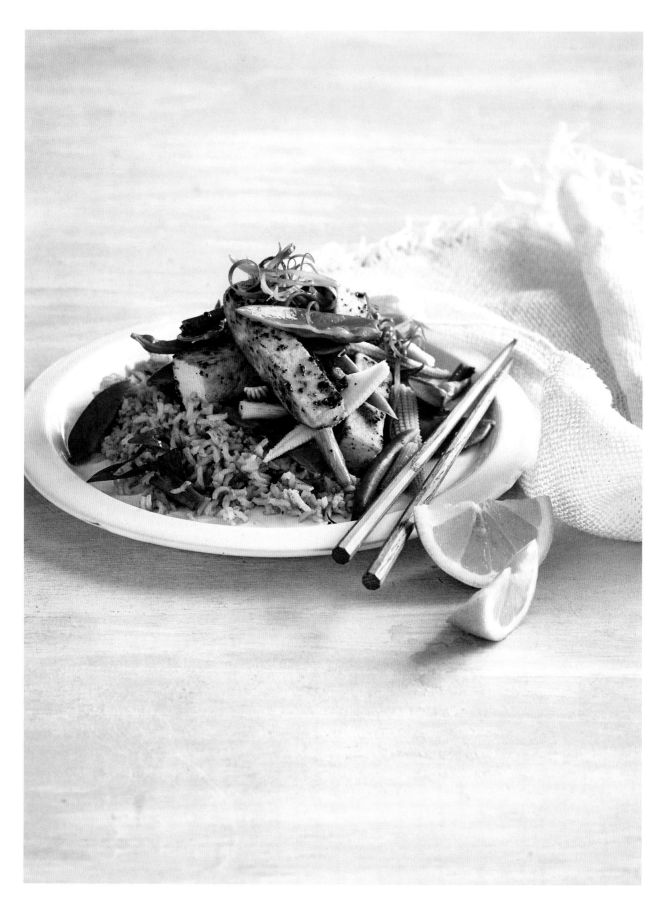

Lemon pepper fried tofu

Preparation: 15 minutes, plus resting time * **Cooking:** 15 minutes
Difficulty: Easy

A

SERVES 4

⅔ cup (140 g) brown basmati rice
2 cups (500 ml) salt-reduced
   vegetable stock
125 g baby corn, halved lengthways
200 g baby green beans, trimmed
150 g snowpeas, trimmed
1 tablespoon sunflower oil
680 g firm tofu, sliced
1 tablespoon lemon pepper seasoning
6 spring onions, white and green parts
   cut into 4 cm lengths
lemon wedges, to serve

Combine the rice and stock in a medium saucepan over high heat and bring to the boil. Immediately reduce the temperature to the lowest possible setting on the smallest stovetop element, then cover and simmer very gently for 15 minutes or until just tender and all the stock has been absorbed. Place the baby corn on top of the rice in the pan, followed by the beans, then the snowpeas. Remove from the heat, cover and leave to stand for 5 minutes.

Meanwhile, heat the sunflower oil in a large, deep non-stick frying pan over high heat. Season the tofu slices on all sides with the lemon pepper seasoning, then fry in the oil for 1–2 minutes or until heated through, crisp and golden. Add the spring onion and cook, tossing gently, for 1 minute or until just wilted.

Divide the rice and vegetables among serving bowls. Top with the tofu mixture and serve with lemon wedges.

UNITS PER SERVE Grains **1** * Meat and alternatives **1** * Fruit **0** * Vegetables **2** * Dairy **0** * Fats and oils **1**

Lunch **121**

ROAST JACKET POTATO WITH FILLINGS

B

All recipes serve 1.

Preheat the oven to 200°C (180°C fan-forced). Scrub either a 300 g potato or a 300 g sweet potato and roast for 45–55 minutes or until a skewer is easily inserted in the centre. Transfer to a plate. Score a cross in the top of the potato or cut the sweet potato down the centre, then ease it open for filling.

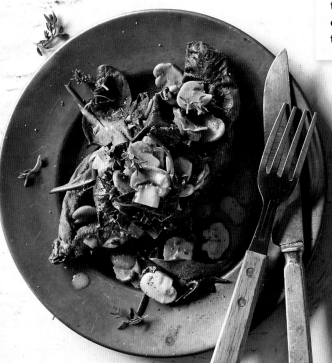

Spinach, ricotta and almond

Combine 120 g fresh reduced-fat ricotta, 2 tablespoons white wine vinegar, 7 g chopped toasted slivered almonds, 1 tablespoon finely chopped chives and ½ teaspoon sweet paprika in a bowl. Season to taste with freshly ground black pepper and set aside. Pour ⅓ cup (80 ml) salt-reduced vegetable stock into a frying pan and bring to the boil over high heat. Add the thinly sliced white part of ½ leek and cook for 3 minutes or until softened and the stock has reduced by two-thirds. Add 2 cups (60 g) shredded English spinach leaves and cook, tossing, for 1 minute or until wilted. Spoon the ricotta mixture into the potato and top with the spinach mixture. Garnish with flat-leaf parsley and season with freshly ground black pepper.

UNITS PER SERVE

Grains **2** ✳ Meat and alternatives **0**
Fruit **0** ✳ Vegetables **2** ✳ Dairy **1**
Fats and oils **1**

Creamy garlic mushroom

Combine 2 teaspoons light margarine, 150 g sliced mushrooms, 1 clove crushed garlic and 2 teaspoons thyme leaves in a small saucepan and cook over medium heat for 30 seconds. Add ½ cup (125 ml) evaporated skim milk and simmer for 8–10 minutes or until the sauce has reduced by about two-thirds. Remove from the heat and stir through 2 cups (60 g) baby spinach leaves until wilted. Season with freshly ground black pepper. Spoon the sauce into the potato and garnish with thyme.

UNITS PER SERVE

Grains **2** ✳ Meat and alternatives **0** ✳ Fruit **0**
Vegetables **2** ✳ Dairy **1** ✳ Fats and oils **1**

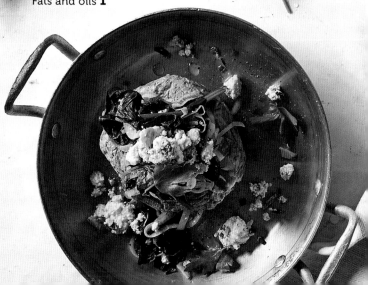

Balsamic onion, asparagus and feta

Melt 2 teaspoons light margarine in a small saucepan over low–medium heat, then add ½ thinly sliced small onion and 1 clove crushed garlic and cook for 10 minutes. Add 1 tablespoon balsamic vinegar and cook for 1 minute. Remove the pan from the heat and stir in 1 bunch trimmed and thinly sliced asparagus. Spoon into the potato, then top with 80 g crumbled reduced-fat feta and ¼ cup small basil leaves. Season with freshly ground black pepper.

UNITS PER SERVE

Grains **2** * Meat and alternatives **0** * Fruit **0**
Vegetables **2** * Dairy **1** * Fats and oils **1**

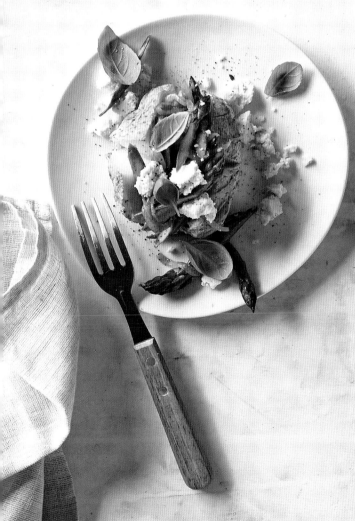

Grilled vegetables with spiced yoghurt

Stir 2 teaspoons Mexican spice mix into 200 g low-fat natural Greek-style yoghurt and set aside. Heat a chargrill pan over high heat, add 1 sliced small zucchini and 2 sliced baby (finger) eggplants and cook for 3 minutes or until just tender. Spoon the vegetables onto the potato, then top with 20 g cubed avocado and ⅓ cup coriander sprigs. Serve with lime wedges and spiced yoghurt.

UNITS PER SERVE

Grains **2** * Meat and alternatives **0** * Fruit **0**
Vegetables **4** * Dairy **1** * Fats and oils **1**

Haloumi and sprout quinoa with spiced yoghurt

Preparation: 20 minutes ✳ **Cooking:** 20 minutes
Difficulty: Easy

B

200 g low-fat natural Greek-style yoghurt
1 tablespoon peri peri sauce
2 tablespoons finely chopped chives
1 cup (190 g) quinoa, well rinsed
light olive oil spray, for cooking
280 g haloumi, thickly sliced (see Notes)
4 medium yellow squash, thickly
    sliced into rounds
1 red onion, sliced into rings
300 g Brussels sprouts, trimmed
    and very thinly sliced
4 red radishes, very thinly
    sliced into rounds
28 g slivered almonds, toasted
mint leaves and lemon wedges, to serve

Preheat a large chargrill pan over high heat.

Combine the yoghurt, peri peri sauce and chives in a bowl. Cover and chill until ready to serve.

Cook the quinoa in a saucepan of boiling water over high heat for 15–18 minutes or until tender. Drain well, then transfer to a large heatproof bowl.

Meanwhile, lightly spray the haloumi, squash and onion on all sides with olive oil. Chargrill, in batches, for 2–3 minutes or until tender and golden.

Divide the quinoa and sprouts amongst four serving bowls. Lay the chargrilled haloumi, vegetables and radish on top and season with freshly ground black pepper. Sprinkle over the almonds and mint leaves and serve with the peri peri yoghurt and lemon wedges alongside.

NOTES

If you want to reduce the salt content of the haloumi, place the slices in a bowl of water for 30 minutes to steep. Drain before use.

UNITS PER SERVE Grains **2** ✳ Meat and alternatives **0** ✳ Fruit **0** ✳ Vegetables **2.5** ✳ Dairy **2** ✳ Fats and oils **1**

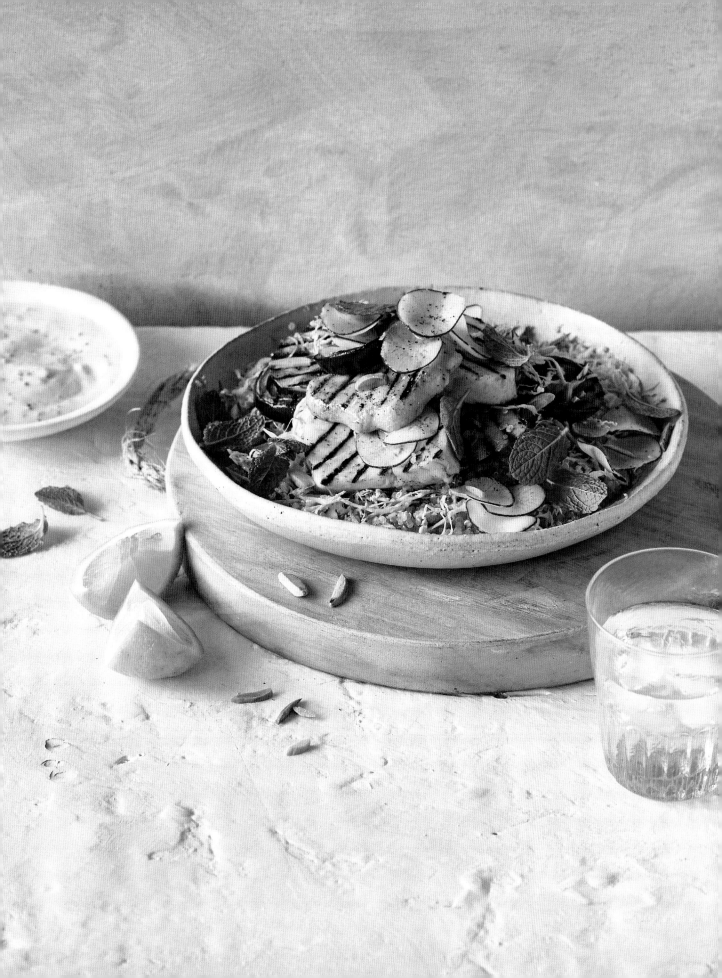

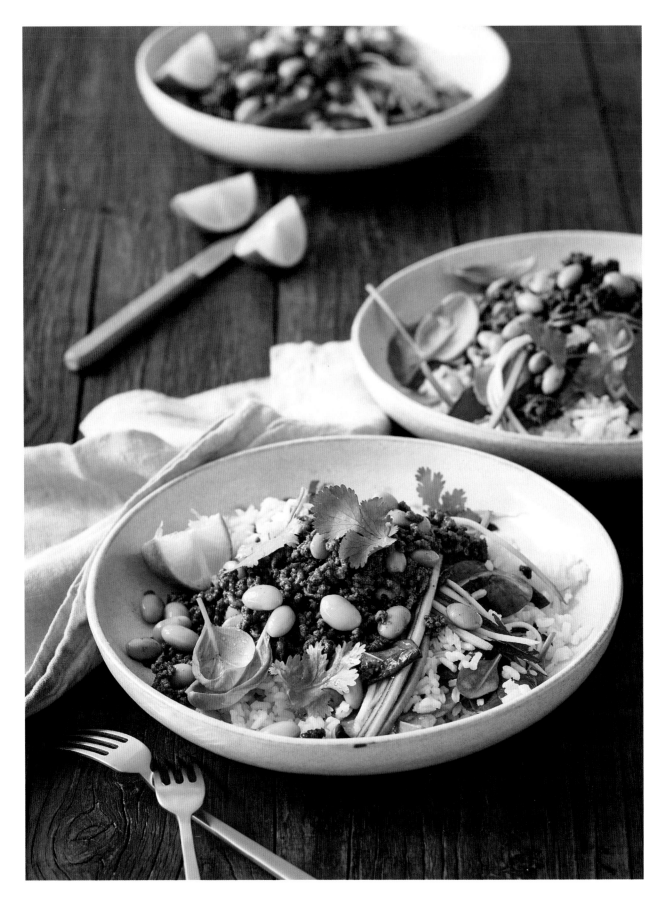

Five-spice beef and green rice

Preparation: 15 minutes * **Cooking:** 25 minutes
Difficulty: Easy

A

¾ cup (160 g) long-grain white rice
1 tablespoon sunflower oil
200 g extra lean minced beef
2 teaspoons five-spice seasoning
300 g frozen shelled edamame,
    thawed (see Notes)
1 tablespoon chilli sauce (optional)
2 cloves garlic, crushed
3 zucchini, peeled into long thin ribbons
3 cups (90 g) baby spinach leaves
½ cup small basil leaves
½ cup small coriander sprigs
lime wedges, to serve

Cook the rice in a large saucepan of boiling water over high heat for 12 minutes or until just tender. Drain and rinse under cold running water, then drain again and set aside.

Heat half the sunflower oil in a large non-stick frying pan over high heat. Add the beef and five-spice seasoning and cook, stirring and breaking up any large lumps with the back of a spoon, for 10 minutes or until cooked and golden. Add the edamame, chilli sauce (if using) and ¼ cup (60 ml) water. Cook, stirring occasionally, for 2 minutes or until the beans are heated through and the water has evaporated.

Meanwhile, heat the remaining sunflower oil in a large wok over high heat. Add the garlic and stir-fry for 2 minutes or until just tender and light golden. Add the zucchini, spinach and drained rice and cook, tossing, for 2 minutes or until the zucchini and spinach have wilted and the rice is hot. Remove the wok from the heat and toss through the basil and coriander.

Divide the green rice among serving bowls and top with the beef mixture. Serve hot with lime wedges.

NOTES

You can find packets of shelled edamame in the freezer section of larger supermarkets and Asian grocers. If unavailable, buy frozen edamame pods and thaw before removing the beans – you will need about 400 g of the pods to yield the quantity of beans required in this recipe.

 MAKE IT VEGETARIAN

Replace the beef mince with vegetarian mince.

UNITS PER SERVE Grains **1** * Meat and alternatives **1** * Fruit **0** * Vegetables **2** * Dairy **0** * Fats and oils **1**

Lunch **127**

Vietnamese prawn vermicelli

Preparation: 20 minutes, plus standing time ✳ **Cooking:** 5 minutes
Difficulty: Medium

A

SERVES 4

1 tablespoon white wine vinegar

1 teaspoon fish sauce

1 tablespoon salt-reduced soy sauce

1 teaspoon ground white pepper

2 teaspoons chilli sauce (optional)

1 red onion, thinly sliced into wedges

1 telegraph cucumber, halved lengthways
    and seeds scraped, thickly sliced

250 g cherry tomatoes, quartered

100 g rice vermicelli

boiling water, for soaking

1 tablespoon sunflower oil

400 g peeled and deveined raw
    medium king prawns

2 cloves garlic, thinly sliced

2 teaspoons finely chopped ginger

½ cup small mint leaves

Using a fork, whisk together the vinegar, fish sauce, soy sauce, pepper, chilli sauce (if using), onion, cucumber and tomato in a large heatproof bowl. Set aside, tossing occasionally.

Place the vermicelli in a large heatproof bowl, cover with boiling water and leave to stand for 5 minutes or until softened. Drain, then rinse under cold running water. Drain again very well, then add to the tomato mixture in the bowl and toss to combine.

Heat the sunflower oil in a large wok over high heat. Add the prawns, garlic and ginger and stir-fry for 3–4 minutes or until the prawns are cooked through. Immediately transfer the prawn mixture to the bowl with the noodles and toss well to combine. Transfer to a serving platter, scatter over the mint leaves and serve warm.

 MAKE IT VEGETARIAN

Replace the fish sauce with tamari. Make a 2-egg omelette and shred finely. Replace the prawns with 500 g diced tofu and cook with the garlic and ginger. Scatter the shredded omelette over the finished dish.

UNITS PER SERVE Grains **1** ✳ Meat and alternatives **1** ✳ Fruit **0** ✳ Vegetables **2.5** ✳ Dairy **0** ✳ Fats and oils **1**

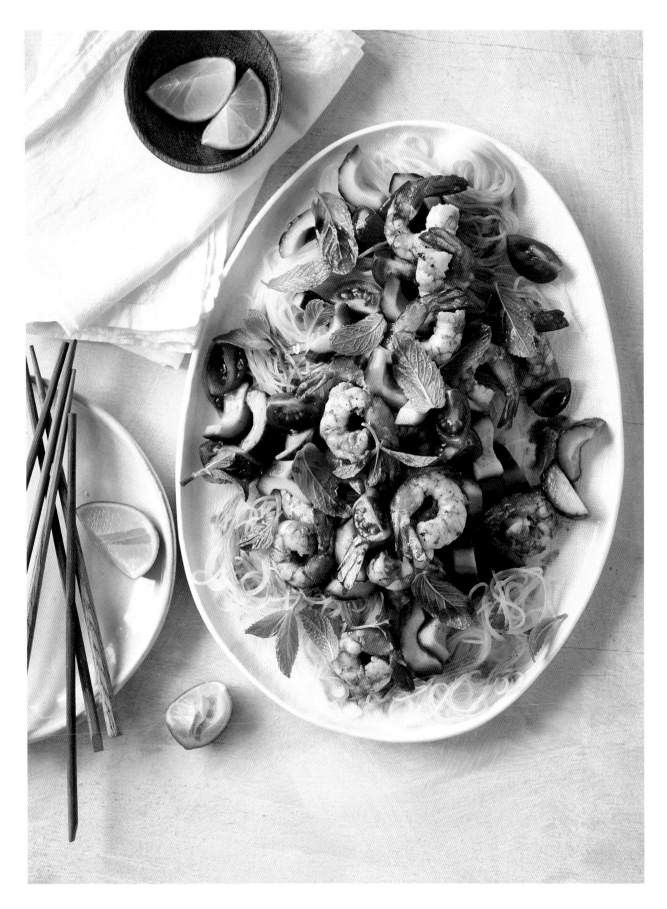

Bocconcini and fresh tomato pasta

Preparation: 15 minutes ✳ **Cooking:** 10 minutes
Difficulty: Easy

B

SERVES 4

1 tablespoon extra virgin olive oil
¼ cup (60 ml) balsamic vinegar
1 clove garlic, crushed
4 tomatoes, chopped
1 x 280 g jar 99% fat-free artichoke hearts
    in brine, drained and halved
1 cup (180 g) chargrilled eggplant slices
    (see Notes), sliced into strips
1 cup small basil leaves
½ cup small flat-leaf parsley leaves
2 cups (400 g) dried wholemeal penne
320 g cherry bocconcini, torn in half

Combine the olive oil, vinegar, garlic, tomato, artichokes, eggplant, basil and parsley in a large heatproof bowl. Season to taste with freshly ground black pepper and set aside.

Cook the pasta in a large saucepan of boiling water over high heat for 8–10 minutes or until just tender. Drain well.

Immediately add the hot pasta to the tomato mixture and toss well to combine. Add the bocconcini and toss again. Serve hot, warm or at room temperature.

NOTES

You can purchase chargrilled eggplant slices from the deli counter of supermarkets. To make your own, slice 1 eggplant into thin rounds and chargrill over high heat for 2–3 minutes each side or until soft.

You can make a double batch of this recipe and store it in an airtight container in the fridge for up to 3 days. It's delicious served straight from the fridge as a cold salad and transports well in an airtight container.

UNITS PER SERVE Grains **2** ✳ Meat and alternatives **0** ✳ Fruit **0** ✳ Vegetables **2.5** ✳ Dairy **2** ✳ Fats and oils **1**

Curried paneer

SERVES 4

1⅓ cups (280 g) brown basmati rice
1 tablespoon sunflower oil
3 teaspoons curry powder
1 large red onion, thinly sliced
680 g paneer, cut into 2 cm pieces
300 g peeled, seeded butternut
    pumpkin, chopped
1 x 400 g tin crushed tomatoes
½ cup (125 ml) salt-reduced
    vegetable stock
1 bunch English spinach, leaves picked
    and well washed

Cook the rice in a large saucepan of boiling water over high heat for 12–15 minutes or until tender. Drain well and keep warm.

Meanwhile, heat the sunflower oil in a large, deep non-stick frying pan over medium–high heat. Add the curry powder and onion and cook, stirring occasionally, for 3 minutes. Add the paneer and pumpkin and cook, stirring occasionally, for a further 3 minutes.

Reduce the heat to low–medium. Add the tomatoes and stock and cook, partially covered and stirring occasionally, for 10 minutes. Remove the lid, stir through the spinach leaves and cook for 2–3 minutes or until the leaves have wilted and all the vegetables are tender.

Divide the rice among serving bowls and spoon over the curry.
Serve hot.

UNITS PER SERVE Grains **2** ❋ Meat and alternatives **0** ❋ Fruit **0** ❋ Vegetables **3** ❋ Dairy **2** ❋ Fats and oils **1**

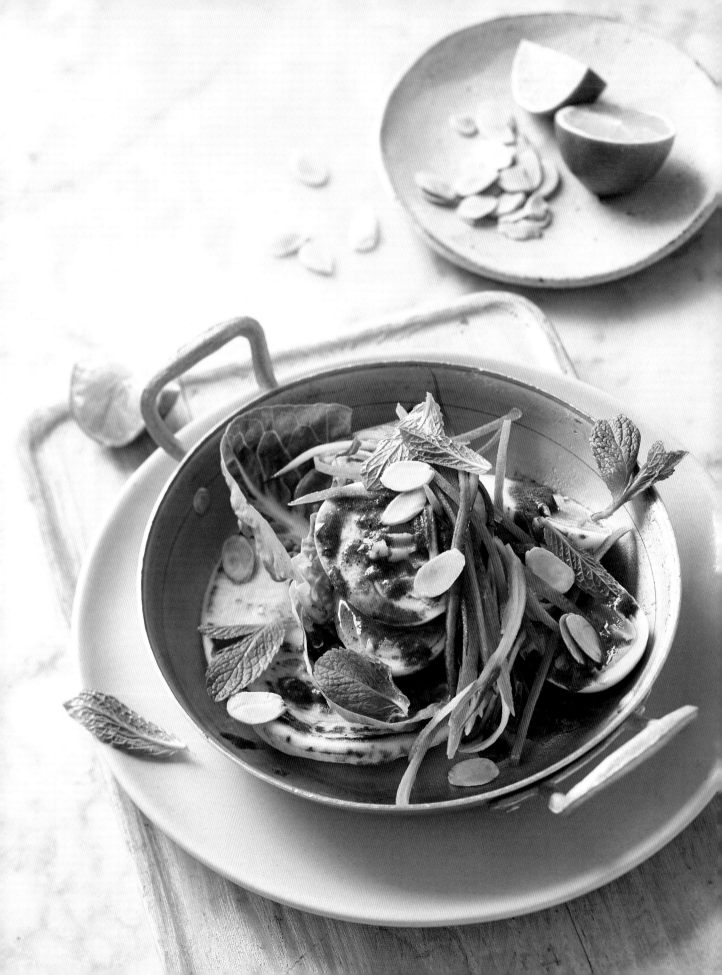

Tikka eggs with naan salad

Preparation: 20 minutes, plus cooling time ✳ **Cooking:** 6 minutes
Difficulty: Easy

A

SERVES 4

2 tablespoons tikka masala
    curry paste
¼ cup (60 ml) white wine vinegar
8 large eggs
1 carrot, peeled into long thin ribbons
1 Lebanese cucumber, peeled into
    long thin ribbons
½ cup small mint leaves
2 tablespoons finely chopped chives
14 g flaked almonds, toasted
4 x 40 g mini naan breads, toasted
1 baby cos lettuce, leaves separated

Using a fork, whisk the curry paste and vinegar in a large heatproof bowl.

Cook the eggs in a large saucepan of boiling water for 6 minutes, then drain. While still hot, carefully remove the shells and cut the eggs in half lengthways. Add to the vinegar mixture in the bowl and very gently toss to coat. Set aside to cool.

Combine the carrot, cucumber, mint, chives and almonds in a bowl and season with freshly ground black pepper.

Divide the naan and cos leaves among serving plates. Top with the tikka eggs, then the carrot mixture and serve.

UNITS PER SERVE Grains **1** ✳ Meat and alternatives **1** ✳ Fruit **0** ✳ Vegetables **2** ✳ Dairy **0** ✳ Fats and oils **1**

Loaded sweet potato wedges

Preparation: 20 minutes ☀ **Cooking:** 50 minutes
Difficulty: Easy

B

SERVES 4

1.2 kg orange sweet potato, skins
   scrubbed, cut into 2 cm thick wedges
light olive oil spray, for cooking
1 x 30 g sachet salt-reduced
   taco seasoning
280 g tasty cheese, coarsely grated
4 ripe tomatoes, finely chopped
1 green capsicum, seeded and
   coarsely chopped
80 g avocado, chopped
2 spring onions, white and green
   parts thinly sliced
juice of ½ lime
½ cup (120 g) low-fat natural
   Greek-style yoghurt
1 long red chilli, seeded and thinly sliced
lime wedges, to serve

Preheat the oven to 200°C (180°C fan-forced). Line a large baking tray with baking paper.

Place the sweet potato wedges on the prepared tray. Lightly spray with olive oil, sprinkle with the taco seasoning and toss well to coat on all sides. Bake for 40 minutes, turning once, until tender.

Sprinkle the cheese over the wedges and bake for a further 10 minutes or until the cheese is melted and bubbling.

Meanwhile, combine the tomato, capsicum, avocado, spring onion and lime juice in a bowl. Season with freshly ground black pepper.

Spoon the tomato mixture over the potatoes. Top with yoghurt and chilli and serve hot with lime wedges.

UNITS PER SERVE Grains **2** ☀ Meat and alternatives **0** ☀ Fruit **0** ☀ Vegetables **3** ☀ Dairy **2** ☀ Fats and oils **1**

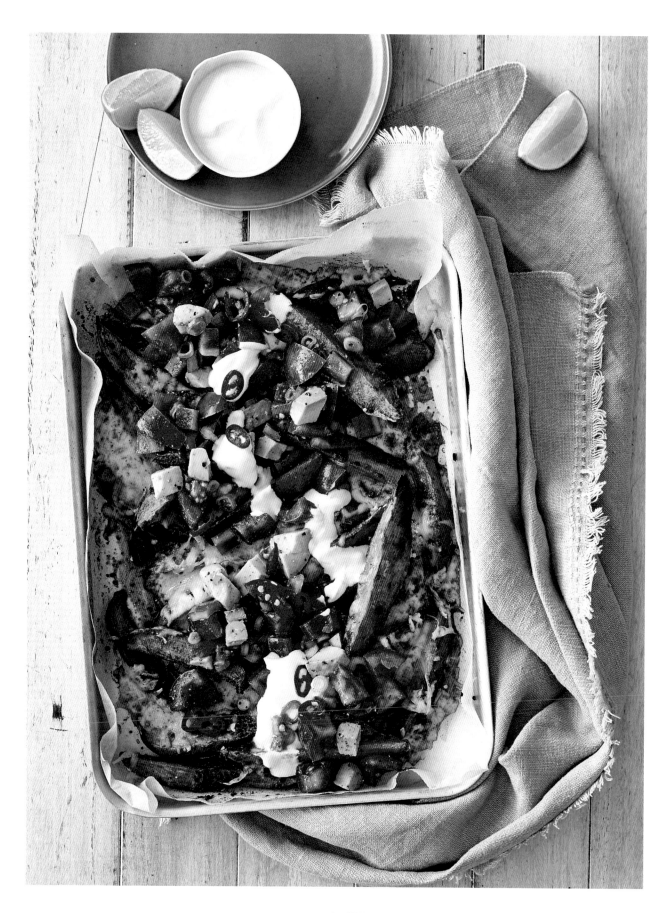

GRAB-AND-GO SNACKS

These simple, throw-together snacks are high in protein and will curb hunger pangs between meals. They use foods from the core food groups, such as fruit and dairy (which would come from your daily allocation if you are following the meal plan), along with grains, healthy fats and oils and vegetables. They are suitable for people who are trying to maintain their weight rather than those following the weight-loss meal plan.

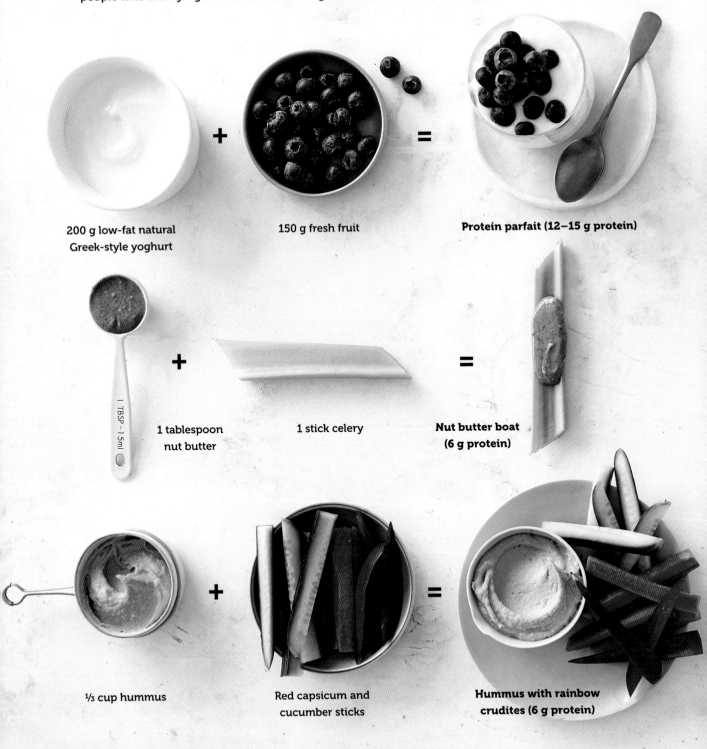

200 g low-fat natural Greek-style yoghurt + 150 g fresh fruit = **Protein parfait (12–15 g protein)**

1 tablespoon nut butter + 1 stick celery = **Nut butter boat (6 g protein)**

⅓ cup hummus + Red capsicum and cucumber sticks = **Hummus with rainbow crudites (6 g protein)**

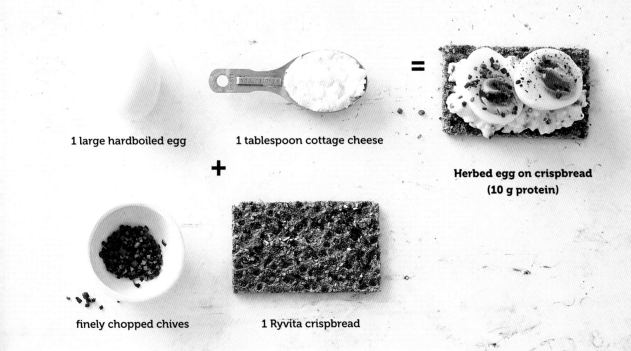

1 large hardboiled egg

+

1 tablespoon cottage cheese

=

**Herbed egg on crispbread
(10 g protein)**

finely chopped chives

1 Ryvita crispbread

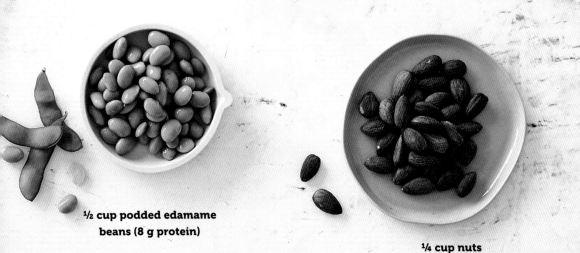

**½ cup podded edamame
beans (8 g protein)**

**¼ cup nuts
(6 g protein)**

Are nuts a good source of protein?
Nuts make a convenient snack and are a good source of protein. They are also a great source of heart-healthy unsaturated fats, and research consistently shows that nuts are an important aspect of a healthy dietary pattern. Because of their high fat content, they are also high in kilojoules (energy), so a small handful is a sensible portion size. The nuts highest in protein are peanuts, followed by almonds and pistachios.

SNACKS TO MAKE AHEAD AND CHILL

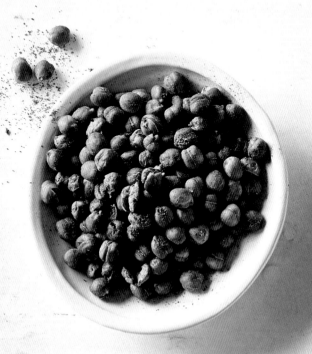

High protein guacamole
Serves 4 / 6.5 g protein per serve

Using a fork, mash together 1 medium (160 g) ripe avocado, ⅔ cup (160 g) low-fat cottage cheese, 2 finely sliced spring onions, 1 large pinch chilli powder and the juice of ½ lemon. Season to taste with freshly ground black pepper and serve immediately with extra finely sliced spring onion to garnish, and ½ cup raw vegetable sticks (such as carrot, cucumber, celery and red capsicum) per person, or store in airtight containers in the fridge for up to 2 days.

Roasted chickpeas
Serves 2 / 8.5 g protein per serve

Preheat the oven to 180°C (160°C fan-forced) and line a large baking tray with baking paper. Drain and rinse a 400 g tin of chickpeas, then pat dry with paper towel. Place the chickpeas in a bowl and add 1 tablespoon mild curry powder, tossing well to coat. Spread chickpeas evenly over the prepared tray and bake for 45 minutes or until golden and crisp. Remove from the oven and leave to cool on the tray. These can be stored in an airtight container for up to 2 days.

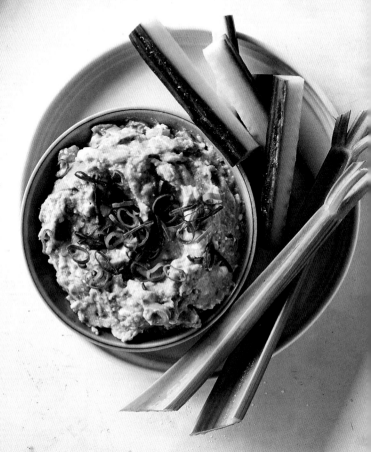

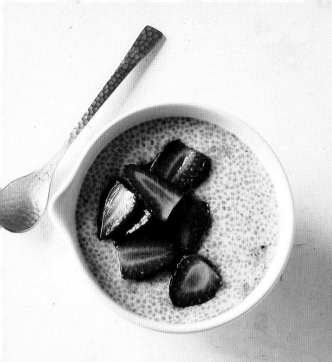

Jaffa protein balls
Makes 16 / 4.5 g protein per ball

Finely grate the zest of 1 large orange and set aside. Juice the orange and place the juice in a small saucepan, along with 20 chopped, pitted dried dates. Place over low heat for a few minutes until the mixture starts to simmer. Remove the pan from the heat and set aside to cool to room temperature, before mashing the mixture together with a fork. Blend 320 g whole natural almonds in a food processor until finely chopped. Add 50 g vanilla protein powder, ¼ cup cocoa powder (reserving 1 tablespoon to dust), 2 teaspoons vanilla, the orange zest and the cooled date mixture, and process until well combined. Roll into 16 balls, dust with the reserved cocoa and place in an airtight container in the fridge to chill before serving. These will keep in the fridge for up to 2 weeks.

Chia puddings with maple strawberries
Serves 2 / 6.5 g protein per serve

Start this the day before you wish to serve it. Whisk 2 tablespoons chia seeds into 200 ml low-fat milk. Set aside for 2 minutes, then whisk again before dividing the mixture between two small serving glasses or cups. Cover and place in the fridge. Hull and halve 125 g small strawberries and place in a bowl with 1 teaspoon pure maple syrup, 1 teaspoon vanilla and ½ teaspoon mixed spice. Stir gently, then cover and place in the fridge with the chia puddings. Leave overnight to allow the fruit to macerate and the puddings to set. When ready to serve, stir the strawberry mixture before spooning over the puddings.

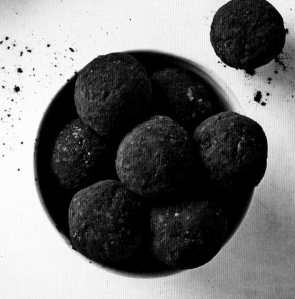

Frozen yoghurt pops
Makes 6 / 7 g protein per serve

Blend 2 cups (500 ml) low-fat natural Greek-style yoghurt, 2 teaspoons honey and 1 cup sliced mixed fruit (such as banana, mango and strawberry) in a food processor until very smooth. Pour into 6 x 180 ml ice-pop moulds or small plastic disposable cups, insert wooden icecream sticks and freeze overnight until firm. These will keep stored in the freezer for up to 1 month.

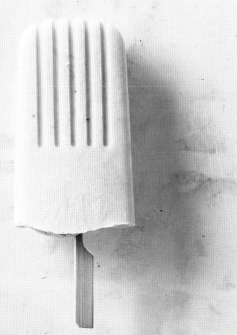

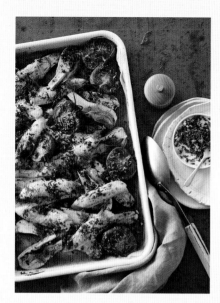

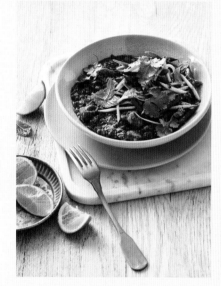

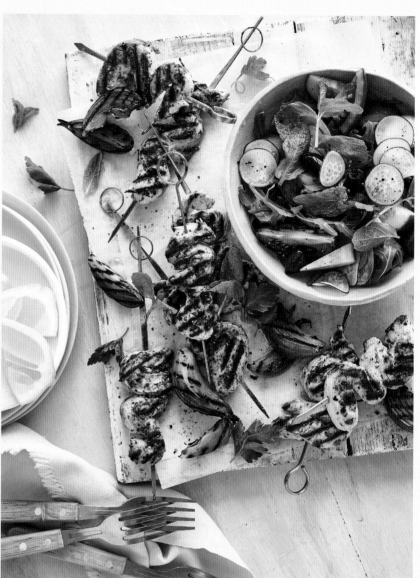

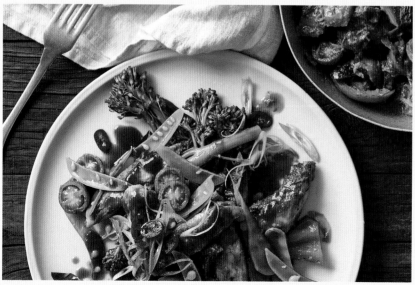

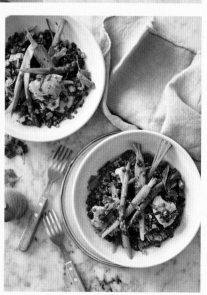

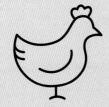

3. Chicken Dinners

Pistachio and herb-topped tenderloins

Preparation: 20 minutes ✳ **Cooking:** 35 minutes
Difficulty: Easy

SERVES 4

4 zucchini, halved lengthways

2 bulbs baby fennel, cut lengthways
  into thirds, green fronds reserved
  for garnish

4 ripe tomatoes, halved horizontally

2 teaspoons fennel seeds

1 teaspoon sweet paprika

½ cup (125 ml) salt-reduced
  chicken stock

light olive oil spray, for cooking

600 g lean chicken tenderloins

28 g unsalted shelled pistachios,
  finely chopped

¼ cup thyme leaves

¼ cup rosemary leaves, finely chopped

¼ cup (60 ml) red wine vinegar

Preheat the oven to 200°C (180°C fan-forced).

Combine the zucchini, fennel, tomatoes, fennel seeds, paprika and stock in a large heavy-based baking dish. Season with freshly ground black pepper and lightly spray with olive oil.

Place the chicken pieces on top of the vegetables and lightly spray with olive oil. Combine the pistachios, thyme and rosemary (reserving a tablespoon for garnish) in a small bowl, then sprinkle over the chicken.

Bake for 30–35 minutes or until the chicken is cooked through. Remove the baking dish from the oven and immediately pour over the vinegar. Serve with the fennel fronds and remaining rosemary scattered on top.

UNITS PER SERVE Grains **0** ✳ Meat and alternatives **1.5** ✳ Fruit **0** ✳ Vegetables **5** ✳ Dairy **0** ✳ Fats and oils **1**

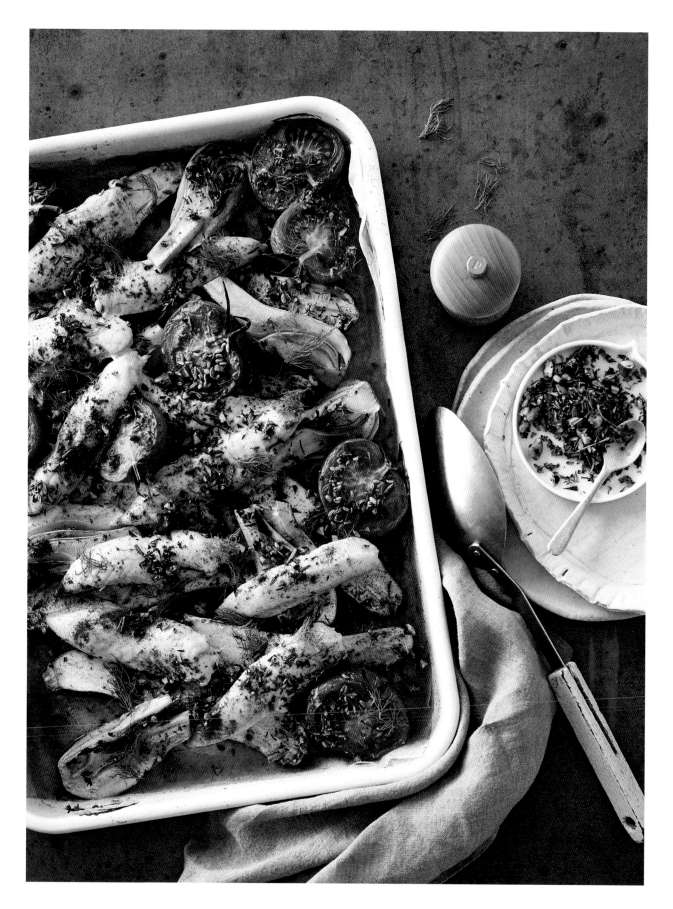

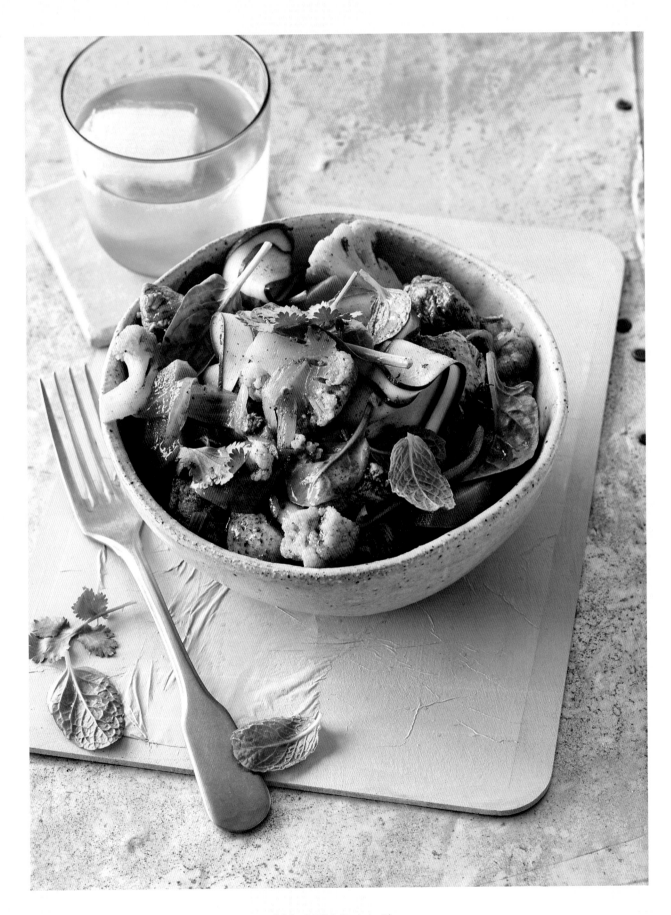

Butter chicken

Preparation: 20 minutes ✳ **Cooking:** 25 minutes
Difficulty: Easy

SERVES 4

2 tablespoons light margarine
1 tablespoon garam masala
2 teaspoons sweet paprika
1 teaspoon ground cinnamon
1 onion, sliced
600 g lean chicken breast fillet,
    cut into 2 cm pieces
3 cups (750 ml) salt-reduced
    chicken stock
4 carrots, chopped
2 cups (200 g) cauliflower florets
2 zucchini, halved lengthways
    and cut into ribbons using
    a vegetable peeler
3 cups (90 g) baby spinach leaves
mint and coriander leaves, to serve

Melt the margarine in a large saucepan over medium heat. Add the spices and onion and cook, stirring occasionally, for 3 minutes, then add the chicken and cook, stirring occasionally, for a further 3 minutes.

Pour in the stock and stir to combine. Add the carrot and cauliflower and cook, stirring occasionally, for 12–15 minutes or until cooked through and the sauce has reduced by half. Add the zucchini ribbons for the last 5 minutes of cooking time. Remove the pan from the heat and stir through the spinach until wilted. Serve scattered with mint and coriander.

UNITS PER SERVE Grains **0** ✳ Meat and alternatives **1.5** ✳ Fruit **0** ✳ Vegetables **3.5** ✳ Dairy **0** ✳ Fats and oils **1**

Baked chicken meatballs

Preparation: 25 minutes * **Cooking:** 40 minutes
Difficulty: Easy

SERVES 4

1 eggplant, chopped

1 large leek, white part only, trimmed then sliced into rounds

1 red capsicum, seeded and sliced

2 x 400 g tins chopped tomatoes

550 g lean minced chicken breast

1 large egg

2 teaspoons dried Italian herbs

1 clove garlic, crushed

2 tablespoons finely chopped chives

2 bunches asparagus, trimmed

1 tablespoon olive oil

Preheat the oven to 200°C (180°C fan-forced).

Combine the eggplant, leek, capsicum and tomatoes in a heavy-based baking dish. Bake for 10 minutes or until hot.

Meanwhile, place the minced chicken, egg, dried herbs, garlic and chives in a large bowl and mix with clean hands until very well combined. Roll the mixture firmly into eight even-sized balls.

Nestle the meatballs into the tomato mixture in the dish and bake for 20 minutes. Remove the dish from the oven. Add the asparagus, drizzle evenly with the olive oil and season with freshly ground black pepper. Return to the oven and bake for a further 10 minutes or until the meatballs are cooked and golden. Take the dish to the table and serve.

UNITS PER SERVE Grains **0** * Meat and alternatives **1.5** * Fruit **0** * Vegetables **5** * Dairy **0** * Fats and oils **1**

Chicken cabbage rolls

Preparation: 25 minutes, plus cooling time ✳ **Cooking:** 1 hour
Difficulty: Medium

SERVES 4

8 large green cabbage leaves,
    thick white core removed
1 tablespoon olive oil
2 cloves garlic, crushed
1 large onion, finely chopped
2 carrots, finely chopped
2 sticks celery, finely chopped
1 teaspoon dried mixed herbs
light olive oil spray, for cooking
600 g lean minced chicken breast
2 x 400 g tins cherry tomatoes
1 cup basil leaves
2 cups (60 g) mixed salad leaves
1 lemon, cut into wedges

Add one cabbage leaf at a time to a large saucepan of boiling water and cook for 1–2 minutes or until just softened and pliable. Drain well and set aside.

Meanwhile, heat the olive oil in a large frying pan over medium heat. Add the garlic, onion, carrot, celery and dried herbs and cook, stirring occasionally, for 5 minutes or until softened and light golden. Transfer to a large bowl and leave to cool.

Preheat the oven to 200°C (180°C fan-forced). Lightly spray a 30 cm x 20 cm baking dish with olive oil.

Add the minced chicken to the cooled vegetable mixture and mix with clean hands until well combined. Season with freshly ground black pepper. Divide the mixture evenly among the softened cabbage leaves, then roll up tightly to form parcels. Place the parcels, seam-side down, in the prepared dish. Pour over the tinned tomatoes to cover.

Cover loosely with foil and bake for 30 minutes. Remove the foil and bake for a further 15 minutes or until the chicken is cooked through and the rolls are caramelised around the edges. Sprinkle with basil and serve hot with salad leaves and lemon wedges.

NOTES

You can swap the tinned cherry tomatoes for the same quantity of tinned chopped tomatoes.

UNITS PER SERVE Grains **0** ✳ Meat and alternatives **1.5** ✳ Fruit **0** ✳ Vegetables **5** ✳ Dairy **0** ✳ Fats and oils **1**

Pepper chilli chicken

Preparation: 15 minutes ✳ **Cooking:** 10 minutes
Difficulty: Easy

SERVES 4

1 tablespoon sunflower oil

1 bunch (3 pieces) baby bok choy,
    leaves separated

600 g lean chicken breast fillet,
    thinly sliced

2 teaspoons freshly ground black pepper

1 red capsicum, seeded and
    roughly chopped

3 carrots, halved lengthways
    and sliced diagonally

2 tablespoons chilli sauce

2 tablespoons salt-reduced soy sauce

1 tablespoon white wine vinegar

2 spring onions, white and green parts
    thinly sliced diagonally

1 long red chilli, thinly sliced into
    matchsticks, to serve (optional)

Heat half the sunflower oil in a large wok over high heat. Add the bok choy and 2 tablespoons water and stir-fry for 2 minutes or until just wilted and light golden. Transfer to serving bowls and cover to keep warm.

Heat the remaining oil in the wok over high heat. Add the chicken and black pepper and stir-fry for 3 minutes. Add all the remaining ingredients, apart from the sliced chilli, and stir-fry for a further 3 minutes or until the chicken is cooked through and the vegetables are just tender.

Spoon the chicken mixture over the bok choy and serve. Garnish with sliced chilli, if using.

UNITS PER SERVE Grains **0** ✳ Meat and alternatives **1.5** ✳ Fruit **0** ✳ Vegetables **3** ✳ Dairy **0** ✳ Fats and oils **1**

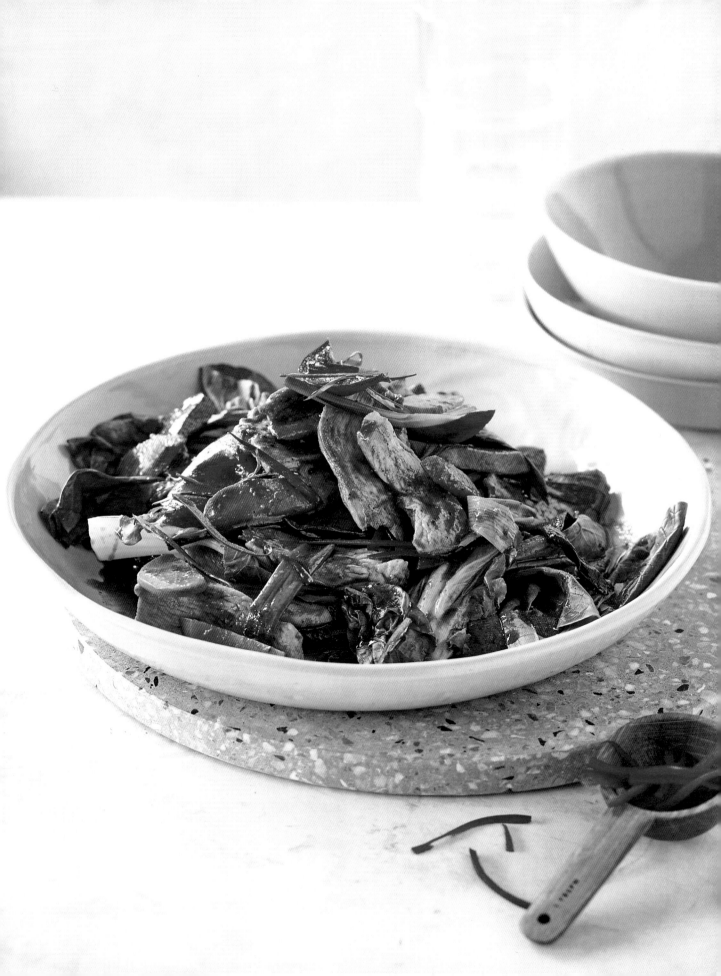

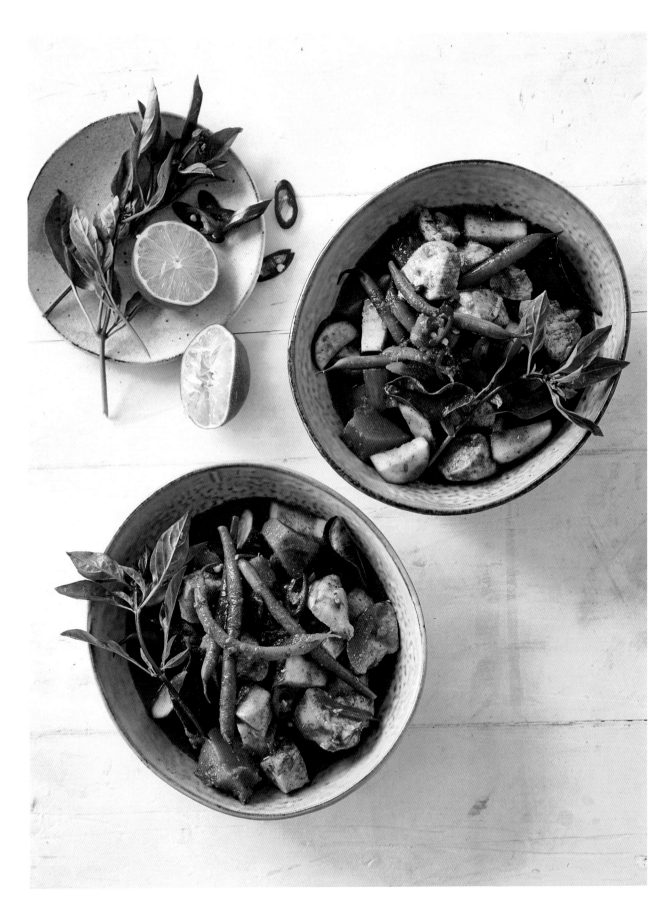

Thai chicken jungle curry

Preparation: 20 minutes * **Cooking:** 15 minutes
Difficulty: Easy

SERVES 4

¼ cup (75 g) Thai red curry paste

2 stalks lemongrass, white part only,
    finely chopped

5 cm piece ginger, cut into
    thin matchsticks

1 large onion, thinly sliced into wedges

600 g lean chicken breast fillet,
    cut into 2 cm pieces

400 g peeled, seeded butternut pumpkin,
    chopped into 2 cm cubes

2 cups (500 ml) salt-reduced
    chicken stock

4 kaffir lime leaves, torn

1 tablespoon tinned green peppercorns
    in brine, drained (see Notes)

2 zucchini, halved lengthways
    and roughly chopped

200 g green beans, trimmed

1 cup Thai basil leaves

1 long red chilli, thinly sliced
    diagonally (optional)

lime wedges, to serve

Heat the curry paste in a large wok over high heat. Add the lemongrass, ginger, onion, chicken and pumpkin and stir-fry for 8 minutes.

Add the stock, lime leaves, peppercorns and zucchini and cook, stirring occasionally, for 5 minutes. Add the beans and cook, tossing gently, for 2 minutes or until the chicken is cooked, the vegetables are just tender and the sauce has reduced slightly.

Divide the chicken curry among serving bowls. Top with the basil and chilli (if using) and serve hot with lime wedges alongside.

NOTES

You will find green peppercorns in the spice aisle of supermarkets, sold in 55 g tins. Leftover peppercorns can be stored, with the brine from the tin, in an airtight container in the fridge for up to 2 weeks.

If you can't find Thai basil, regular basil will work just as well.

UNITS PER SERVE Grains **0** * Meat and alternatives **1.5** * Fruit **0** * Vegetables **3** * Dairy **0** * Fats and oils **1**

MAKE IT THREE WAYS

Save time and money, and reduce food waste, by cooking
once and turning it into three complete meals.

Roast herbed chicken and veg

Preparation: 25 minutes ✳ **Cooking:** 30 minutes
Difficulty: Easy

SERVES 4, WITH LEFTOVERS

½ cup finely chopped flat-leaf parsley
2 tablespoons finely chopped rosemary
1 tablespoon mixed dried herbs
6 cloves garlic, crushed
¼ cup (60 ml) olive oil
¼ cup (60 ml) red wine vinegar
1.8 kg lean chicken tenderloins
1 head cauliflower, cut into florets
7 carrots, sliced into rounds
7 zucchini, thickly sliced into rounds
750 g button mushrooms
light olive oil spray, for cooking
1 cup (250 ml) salt-reduced chicken stock
lemon wedges and flat-leaf parsley
    leaves, to serve

Preheat the oven to 200°C (180°C fan-forced).

Combine the parsley, rosemary, dried herbs, garlic, olive oil, vinegar
and chicken in a large bowl. Season generously with freshly ground
black pepper and toss well to coat the chicken.

Divide the vegetables among two large roasting tins and lightly spray
with olive oil. Toss to combine, then top evenly with the chicken mixture.
Pour half the stock over the ingredients in each tin.

Bake, swapping the tins halfway through and tossing the chicken and
vegetables, for 25–30 minutes or until the chicken is cooked through and
the veggies are soft. Divide one-third of the chicken and vegetables among
four for dinner, with lemon wedges and parsley. Cool the leftovers, then
divide evenly between two large airtight containers.

NOTES

*Store the leftovers in the fridge for up to 2 days or in the freezer for
3 months. Thaw the frozen mixture in the fridge overnight. Transfer
the chilled mixture to a baking dish and reheat in a preheated 220°C
(200°C fan-forced) oven for 15–20 minutes or until hot and crispy.*

UNITS PER SERVE Grains **0** ✳ Meat and alternatives **1.5** ✳ Fruit **0**
Vegetables **3** ✳ Dairy **0** ✳ Fats and oils **1**

USING THE LEFTOVERS...

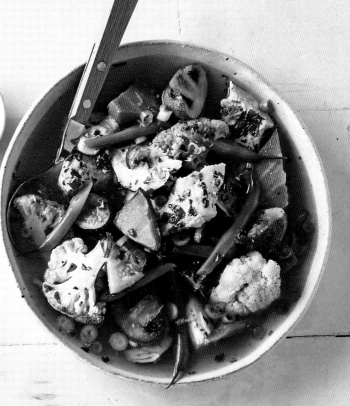

Warm Moroccan chicken and veggie salad

Preparation: 15 minutes * **Cooking:** 20 minutes
Difficulty: Easy

SERVES 4

Take one portion of leftovers and thickly slice the chicken, then place the chicken and vegetables in a large baking dish. Line a baking tray with baking paper. Place 2 red onions, cut into wedges, and 1 punnet cherry tomatoes on the tray. Lightly spray with light olive oil and sprinkle with 1 tablespoon Moroccan spice mix. Place the dish and tray in the oven and bake for 20 minutes. Transfer the tomato and onion to the dish with the chicken and vegetables, add 1 cup (30 g) baby rocket leaves and gently toss to combine. Serve warm.

UNITS PER SERVE Grains **0** * Meat and alternatives **1.5** * Fruit **0** * Vegetables **5** * Dairy **0**
Fats and oils **1**

Hearty chicken soup

Preparation: 15 minutes * **Cooking:** 15 minutes
Difficulty: Easy

SERVES 4

Place the finely grated zest and juice of 1 large lemon, 1 seeded and finely chopped long red chilli, 2 finely chopped spring onions, 2 tablespoons finely chopped coriander and 2 tablespoons finely chopped flat-leaf parsley in a bowl. Mix together well and set aside. Take one portion of leftovers and chop the chicken into bite-sized pieces. Place the chicken and vegetables in a large saucepan, add 1.5 litres salt-reduced chicken stock and bring to a simmer over medium heat. Simmer for 10 minutes or until heated through. Stir in 100 g trimmed and halved baby green beans and cook for 1 minute or until just tender. Ladle into bowls and drizzle with the reserved herb mixture.

UNITS PER SERVE Grains **0** * Meat and alternatives **1.5** * Fruit **0** * Vegetables **3.5** * Dairy **0**
Fats and oils **1**

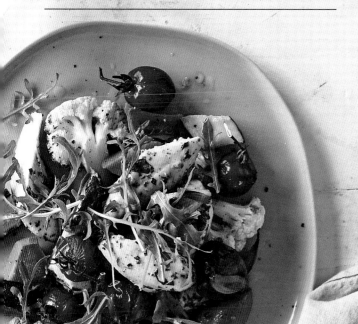

Chicken dhal and herbed greens

Preparation: 20 minutes ✳ **Cooking:** 30 minutes
Difficulty: Easy

SERVES 4

¼ cup (75 g) madras curry paste
1 tablespoon finely chopped ginger
2 cloves garlic, crushed
2 tablespoons salt-reduced tomato paste
1 large red onion, chopped
300 g lean chicken breast fillet,
    cut into 2 cm pieces
¾ cup (140 g) dried split red lentils
1 litre salt-reduced chicken stock
lime wedges, to serve

HERBED GREENS

2 tablespoons white wine vinegar
1 teaspoon wholegrain mustard
200 g green beans, trimmed
    and halved diagonally
2 zucchini, cut into thin matchsticks
½ cup coriander leaves
½ cup small mint leaves
2 spring onions, white and green
    parts thinly sliced

Heat the curry paste in a large heavy-based saucepan over medium heat. Add the ginger, garlic, tomato paste and onion and cook, stirring occasionally, for 5 minutes or until fragrant and the onion is golden. Add the chicken and cook, stirring, for 2 minutes. Add the lentils and stir for 1 minute or until they are well coated in the onion mixture.

Pour in the stock and stir to combine. Reduce the heat to low, then cover and cook, stirring occasionally, for 18–20 minutes or until the chicken is cooked, the lentils are tender and the stock has been completely absorbed. Remove the pan from the heat and season with freshly ground black pepper.

Meanwhile, to make the herbed greens, use a fork to whisk the vinegar and mustard in a large heatproof bowl. Season with freshly ground black pepper and set aside. Cook the beans in a saucepan of boiling water over high heat for 2 minutes or until just tender. Drain well, then immediately add to the mustard mixture in the bowl. Add all the remaining ingredients and toss well to combine.

Divide the chicken dhal among bowls and serve with the herbed greens and lime wedges alongside.

UNITS PER SERVE Grains **0** ✳ Meat and alternatives **1.5** ✳ Fruit **0** ✳ Vegetables **3** ✳ Dairy **0** ✳ Fats and oils **1**

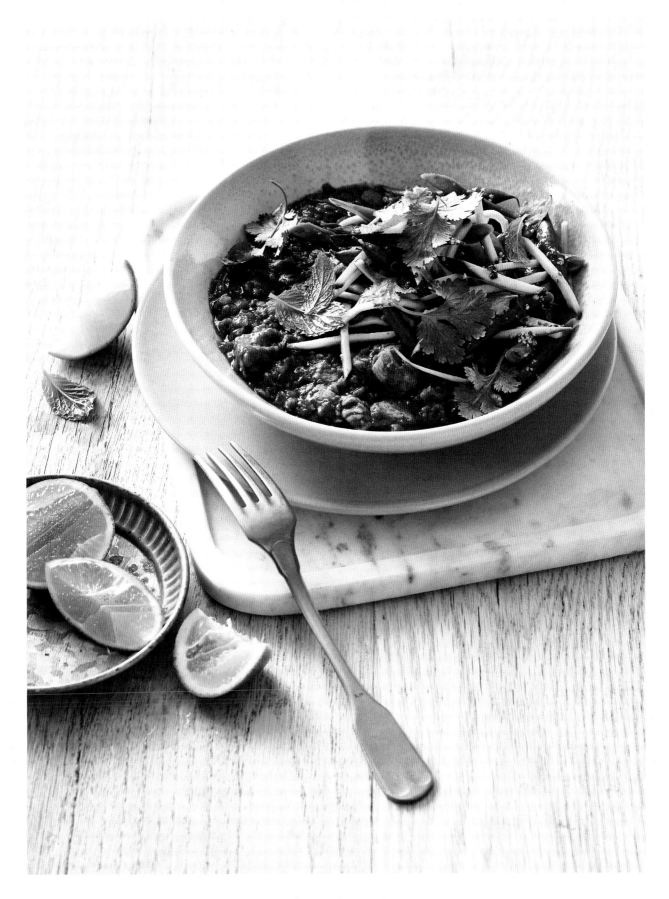

Chicken chow mein

Preparation: 15 minutes ✳ **Cooking:** 10 minutes
Difficulty: Easy

SERVES 4

3 teaspoons sunflower oil

½ teaspoon sesame oil

600 g lean chicken breast fillet,
   thinly sliced

1 onion, thinly sliced

2 cloves garlic, thinly sliced

1 tablespoon finely chopped ginger

¼ cup (60 ml) salt-reduced soy sauce

2 tablespoons salt-reduced oyster sauce

2 carrots, cut into matchsticks

125 g baby corn, halved lengthways

200 g button mushrooms, thickly sliced

400 g green cabbage, shredded

2 spring onions, white and green parts
   cut into 2 cm lengths

Heat the sunflower and sesame oils in a large wok over high heat. Add the chicken, onion, garlic and ginger and stir-fry for 3 minutes.

Add all the remaining ingredients and ¼ cup (60 ml) water and stir-fry for 3–5 minutes or until the chicken is cooked through and the vegetables are tender. Serve hot.

UNITS PER SERVE Grains **0** ✳ Meat and alternatives **1.5** ✳ Fruit **0** ✳ Vegetables **3** ✳ Dairy **0** ✳ Fats and oils **1**

Chicken satay

Preparation: 20 minutes ✻ **Cooking:** 20 minutes
Difficulty: Easy

SERVES 4

600 g lean chicken tenderloins,
    halved lengthways
1 teaspoon ground turmeric
1 teaspoon ground coriander
1 teaspoon ground cumin
light olive oil spray, for cooking
2 telegraph cucumbers, halved
    lengthways and seeds scraped,
    thinly sliced
1 cup (80 g) bean sprouts, trimmed
2 cups (120 g) shredded iceberg lettuce
½ cup small mint leaves

SATAY SAUCE
¼ cup (75 g) Thai yellow curry paste
1 red onion, finely chopped
28 g roasted unsalted peanuts,
    finely chopped
2 teaspoons salt-reduced oyster sauce
1 cup (250 ml) salt-reduced chicken stock

To make the satay sauce, heat the curry paste in a small saucepan over medium heat. Add the onion and cook, stirring occasionally, for 5 minutes or until softened and golden. Add the peanuts, oyster sauce and stock and cook, stirring occasionally, for 5 minutes or until the mixture has reduced by one-third. Cover to keep warm and set aside.

Heat a chargrill pan over high heat. Combine the chicken and spices in a bowl and lightly spray with olive oil. Add to the chargrill pan and cook, turning occasionally, for 5–8 minutes or until cooked and golden.

Meanwhile, combine the cucumber, bean sprouts, lettuce and mint in a bowl.

Divide the cucumber salad among serving plates and place the chicken on top. Spoon over the satay sauce and serve.

🌿 **MAKE IT VEGETARIAN**

Substitute the chicken for 1 kg tofu. Replace the oyster sauce with tamari and use vegetable stock instead of chicken stock.

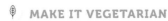

UNITS PER SERVE Grains **0** ✻ Meat and alternatives **1.5** ✻ Fruit **0** ✻ Vegetables **3** ✻ Dairy **0** ✻ Fats and oils **1**

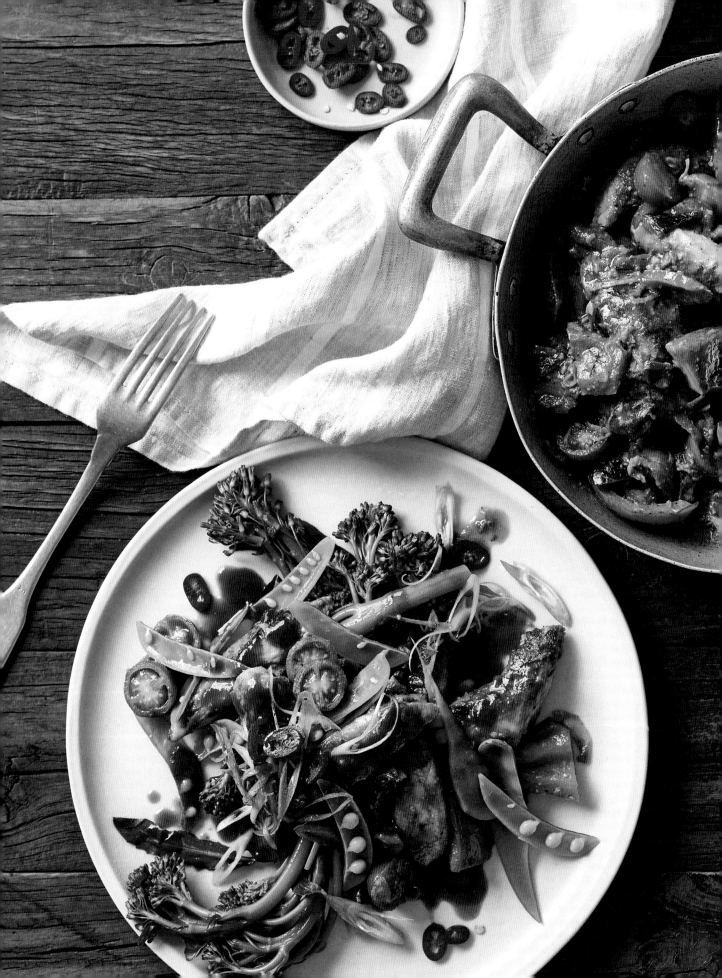

Sweet and sour crunchy chicken

Preparation: 20 minutes * **Cooking:** 10 minutes
Difficulty: Easy

SERVES 4

1 tablespoon cornflour
1 large egg
1 tablespoon salt-reduced soy sauce
550 g lean chicken tenderloins,
    halved diagonally
1 tablespoon sunflower oil
1 large red onion, chopped
3 cloves garlic, crushed
5 cm piece ginger,
    cut into thin matchsticks
1 green capsicum, seeded and chopped
250 g cherry tomatoes, halved
2 tablespoons salt-reduced tomato sauce
1 tablespoon salt-reduced hoisin sauce
1 tablespoon white wine vinegar
3 cups mixed steamed greens
    (such as snowpeas, sugar
    snap peas and broccolini)
finely sliced spring onion and red chilli,
    to serve (optional)

Using a fork, whisk the cornflour, egg and soy sauce in a bowl until well combined. Add the chicken pieces and turn to coat on all sides.

Heat the sunflower oil in a large wok over high heat, add the chicken and stir-fry for 3 minutes or until crispy and light golden. Add the onion, garlic, ginger and capsicum and stir-fry for a further 3 minutes.

Add the tomatoes, tomato sauce, hoisin and vinegar and toss to combine, then immediately remove the wok from the heat.

Divide the steamed vegetables among serving bowls, top with the sweet and sour chicken and serve with finely sliced spring onion and red chilli, if using.

UNITS PER SERVE Grains **0** * Meat and alternatives **1.5** * Fruit **0** * Vegetables **3.5** * Dairy **0** * Fats and oils **1**

Chicken and vegetable 'lasagne'

Preparation: 25 minutes ✳ **Cooking:** 45 minutes
Difficulty: Medium

SERVES 4

light olive oil spray, for cooking
4 large zucchini, thinly sliced lengthways
2 eggplants, thinly sliced into rounds
500 g peeled, seeded butternut pumpkin,
    thinly sliced
600 g lean chicken breast fillet
2 teaspoons dried mixed herbs
700 g tomato passata
2 cups (60 g) baby spinach leaves
28 g flaked almonds
1 bunch rocket, leaves trimmed
2 teaspoons balsamic vinegar

Preheat the oven to 200°C (180°C fan-forced).

Heat a large chargrill pan over high heat. Lightly spray the zucchini, eggplant and pumpkin on both sides with olive oil. Chargrill, in four batches, for 3–4 minutes or until just tender and golden.

Slice the chicken breast in half horizontally, then place the pieces between two sheets of baking paper and pound with a meat mallet until 2 mm thick. Sprinkle with the dried herbs and season with freshly ground black pepper.

Lightly spray a 30 cm x 20 cm baking dish with olive oil. Spoon a little of the passata over the base of the dish. Top with a layer of chicken, some baby spinach leaves and then a layer of chargrilled vegetables. Spoon over more passata to cover evenly, then repeat the layers with the remaining chicken, baby spinach, vegetables and passata, finishing with a final layer of passata. Sprinkle the top with almonds.

Bake for 30 minutes or until the chicken is cooked through and golden. Serve with rocket leaves tossed in balsamic.

UNITS PER SERVE Grains **0** ✳ Meat and alternatives **1.5** ✳ Fruit **0** ✳ Vegetables **8** ✳ Dairy **0** ✳ Fats and oils **1**

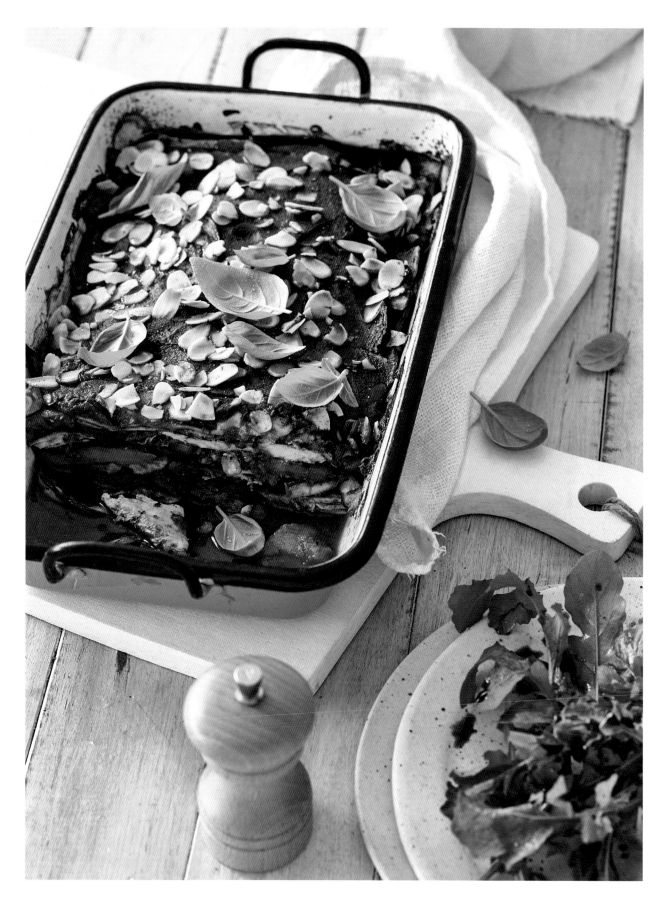

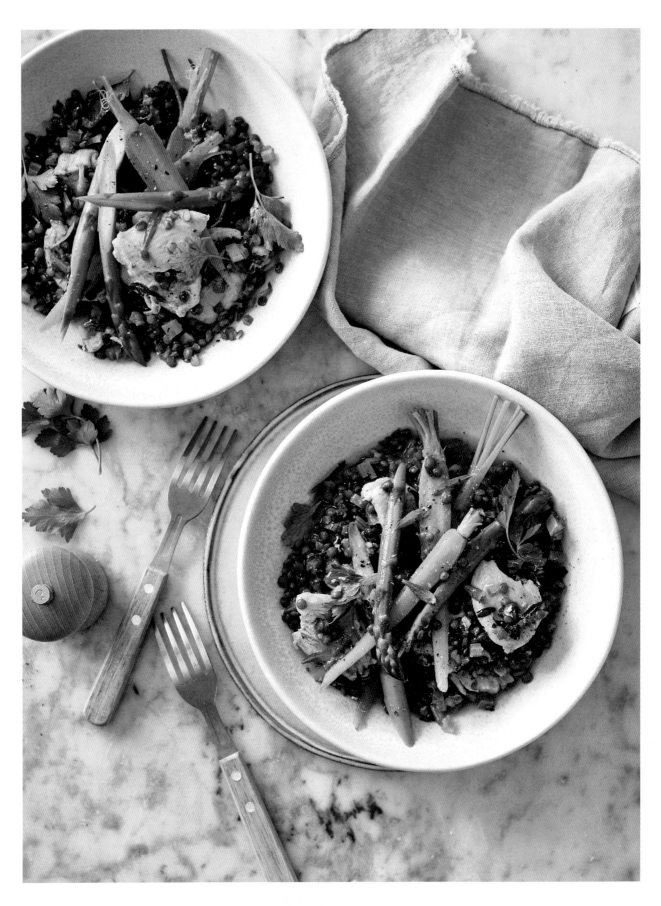

Chicken and lentil braise

Preparation: 20 minutes ✳ **Cooking:** 20 minutes
Difficulty: Easy

SERVES 4

1 tablespoon olive oil

1 large onion, finely chopped

2 sticks celery, finely chopped

2 cloves garlic, crushed

400 g lean chicken breast fillet,
    cut into 2 mm thick slices

2 tablespoons white wine vinegar

2 tablespoons chopped tarragon

300 g drained, rinsed tinned lentils

2 bunches baby carrots, trimmed,
    skins scrubbed, halved lengthways
    or 2 carrots, roughly chopped

2 cups (500 ml) salt-reduced
    chicken stock

1 bunch asparagus, trimmed, cut into
    4 cm lengths on the diagonal

¼ cup small flat-leaf parsley leaves

Heat the olive oil in a large deep frying pan over medium heat. Add the onion, celery and garlic and cook, stirring occasionally, for 5 minutes or until softened and light golden.

Add the chicken, vinegar, tarragon, lentils, carrots and stock and cook, stirring occasionally, for 10 minutes. Add the asparagus and cook, shaking the pan occasionally, for a further 3 minutes or until the chicken is cooked through and the sauce has reduced by half.

Divide the chicken braise among serving bowls, top with parsley leaves and serve.

NOTES

You will need two 400 g tins of lentils for this recipe. Store any leftover lentils in an airtight container in the fridge for up to 3 days or in the freezer for up to 3 months.

UNITS PER SERVE Grains **0** ✳ Meat and alternatives **1.5** ✳ Fruit **0** ✳ Vegetables **3.5** ✳ Dairy **0** ✳ Fats and oils **1**

Greek chicken kebabs

Preparation: 25 minutes, plus chilling time ✳ **Cooking:** 10 minutes
Difficulty: Medium

SERVES 4

1 tablespoon olive oil

2 teaspoons dried oregano

2 cloves garlic, crushed

600 g lean chicken tenderloins,
    halved lengthways

finely grated zest and juice
    of 1 large lemon

1 red onion, cut into wedges

4 tomatoes, cut into wedges

1 telegraph cucumber, halved
    lengthways and thinly sliced

6 radishes, thinly sliced into rounds

2 tablespoons chopped mint

1 cup small flat-leaf parsley leaves

½ cup (75 g) pitted kalamata olives

1 cup (30 g) rocket leaves

Combine the olive oil, oregano, garlic, chicken, lemon zest and half the lemon juice in a non-metallic bowl. Cover and place in the fridge for 20 minutes to marinate. Using 12 metal skewers, thread two pieces of chicken onto each.

Preheat a barbecue chargrill plate to medium–high. Add the skewers and onion wedges and cook, turning occasionally, for 8–10 minutes or until cooked through.

Meanwhile, combine the tomato, cucumber, radish, mint, parsley, olives, rocket and remaining lemon juice in a large bowl. Season with freshly ground black pepper.

Divide the salad among serving plates, add the chicken kebabs and chargrilled onion and serve.

NOTES

You can use a chargrill pan for this recipe if you don't want to fire up the barbecue. Use a large pan and cook the chicken and onion in two batches.

UNITS PER SERVE Grains **0** ✳ Meat and alternatives **1.5** ✳ Fruit **0** ✳ Vegetables **3.5** ✳ Dairy **0** ✳ Fats and oils **1**

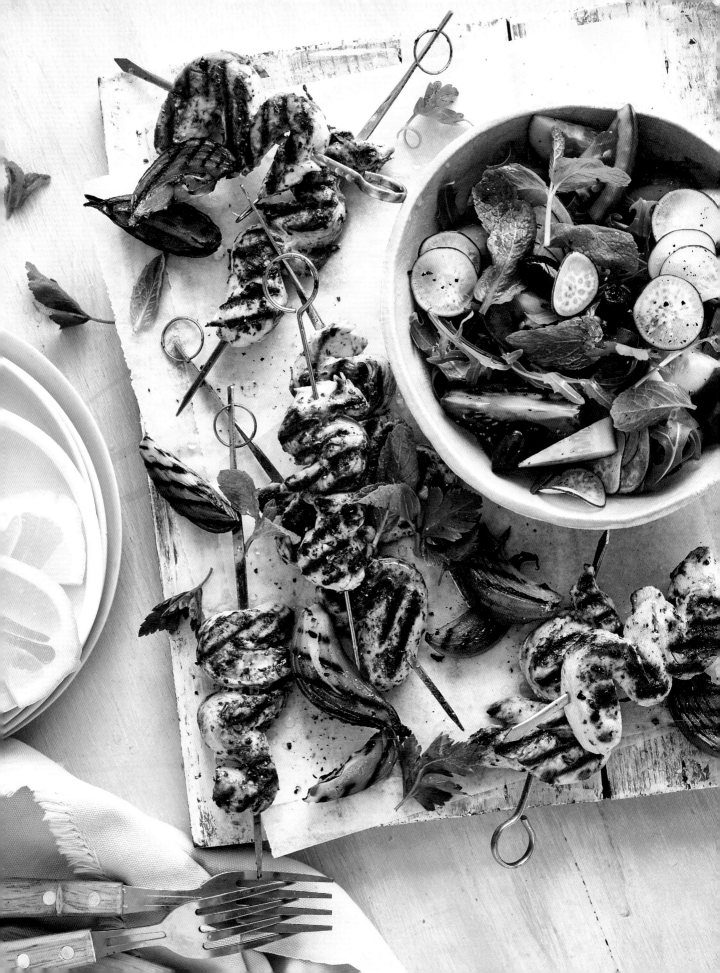

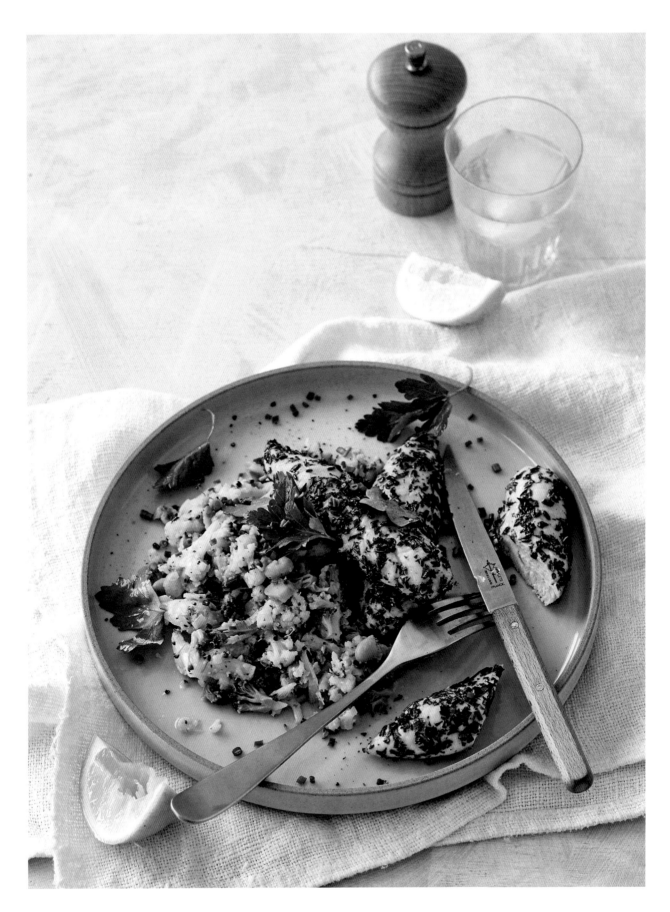

Cumin chicken with cannellini mash

Preparation: 25 minutes ✳ **Cooking:** 15 minutes
Difficulty: Easy

SERVES 4

400 g lean chicken tenderloins

2 tablespoons cumin seeds

2 tablespoons finely chopped
    flat-leaf parsley

2 tablespoons finely chopped chives

2 teaspoons olive oil

1 tablespoon light margarine

1 leek, white part only, thinly
    sliced into rounds

300 g drained, rinsed tinned
    cannellini beans

2 teaspoons wholegrain mustard

2 cups (170 g) broccoli florets

4 cups (400 g) cauliflower florets

1 cup (250 ml) salt-reduced chicken stock

lemon wedges, to serve

flat-leaf parsley leaves, to serve

Preheat the oven grill to high. Combine the chicken, cumin seeds, parsley, chives and 1 teaspoon olive oil in a bowl and season with freshly ground black pepper. Transfer to a large non-stick baking tray in a single layer. Cook under the grill, turning occasionally, for 12–15 minutes or until cooked and golden.

Meanwhile, heat the margarine and remaining olive oil in a large deep frying pan over medium–high heat. Add the leek and cook, stirring occasionally, for 3 minutes or until softened. Add all the remaining ingredients and cook, stirring occasionally, for 8–10 minutes or until the vegetables are tender and the stock has reduced by two-thirds. Remove the pan from the heat and roughly mash the ingredients together.

Divide the cannellini mash among serving plates. Top with the chicken and any tray juices and serve with lemon wedges alongside and parsley sprinkled over the top.

NOTE

You will need two 400 g tins of cannellini beans for this recipe. Store any leftover beans in an airtight container in the fridge for up to 3 days or in the freezer for up to 3 months.

UNITS PER SERVE Grains **0** ✳ Meat and alternatives **1.5** ✳ Fruit **0** ✳ Vegetables **3** ✳ Dairy **0** ✳ Fats and oils **1**

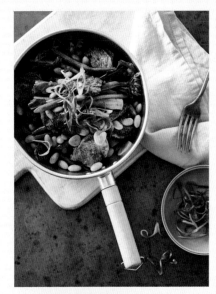

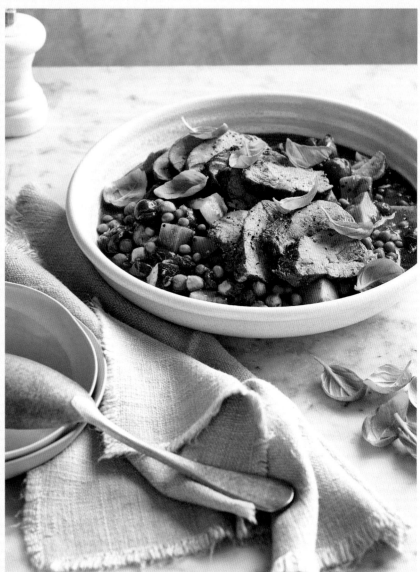

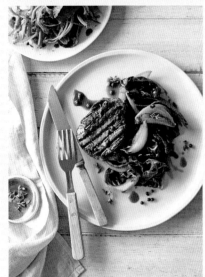

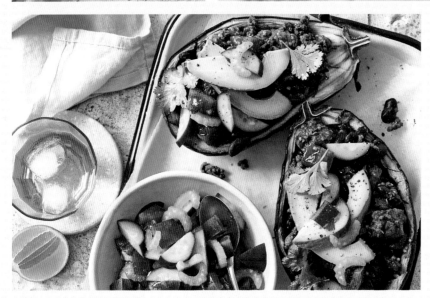

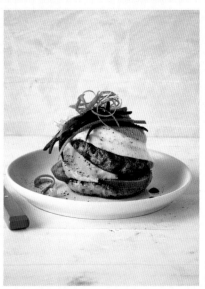

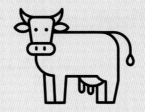

4. Beef, Lamb and Pork Dinners

Beef and black bean stew

Preparation: 15 minutes ✳ **Cooking:** 20 minutes
Difficulty: Easy

SERVES 4

400 g lean minced beef

300 g drained, rinsed tinned black beans

2 tablespoons salt-reduced tomato paste

1 tablespoon sweet paprika

1 red onion, thinly sliced

1 red capsicum, seeded and thinly sliced

1 green capsicum, seeded
    and thinly sliced

1 cup (250 ml) salt-reduced beef stock

4 cobs cooked sweetcorn, husk and
    silks removed, kernels sliced off

80 g avocado, finely chopped

1 long green chilli, seeded
    and thinly sliced

lime wedges, to serve

coriander leaves, to serve

Heat a large, deep non-stick frying pan over high heat. Add the minced beef and cook, stirring and breaking up any lumps with the back of a spoon, for 10 minutes. Add the black beans, tomato paste and paprika and cook, stirring, for 2 minutes or until fragrant.

Reduce the heat to medium. Add the onion and red and green capsicum and cook, stirring occasionally, for 3 minutes. Pour in the stock and cook, stirring occasionally, for 5 minutes or until the vegetables are tender and the stock has reduced by three-quarters.

Meanwhile, combine the corn, avocado and chilli in a bowl. Season with freshly ground black pepper.

Divide the beef stew among serving bowls, top with the corn salsa and serve with lime wedges and coriander.

NOTES

You will need two 400 g tins of black beans for this recipe. Store any leftover beans in an airtight container in the fridge for up to 3 days or in the freezer for up to 3 months. Black beans can be found in the Mexican food section or with the tinned legumes at the supermarket.

 ## MAKE IT VEGETARIAN

Replace the beef mince with the same quantity of vegetarian mince, and use vegetable stock in place of beef stock.

UNITS PER SERVE Grains **0** ✳ Meat and alternatives **1.5** ✳ Fruit **0** ✳ Vegetables **3.5** ✳ Dairy **0** ✳ Fats and oils **1**

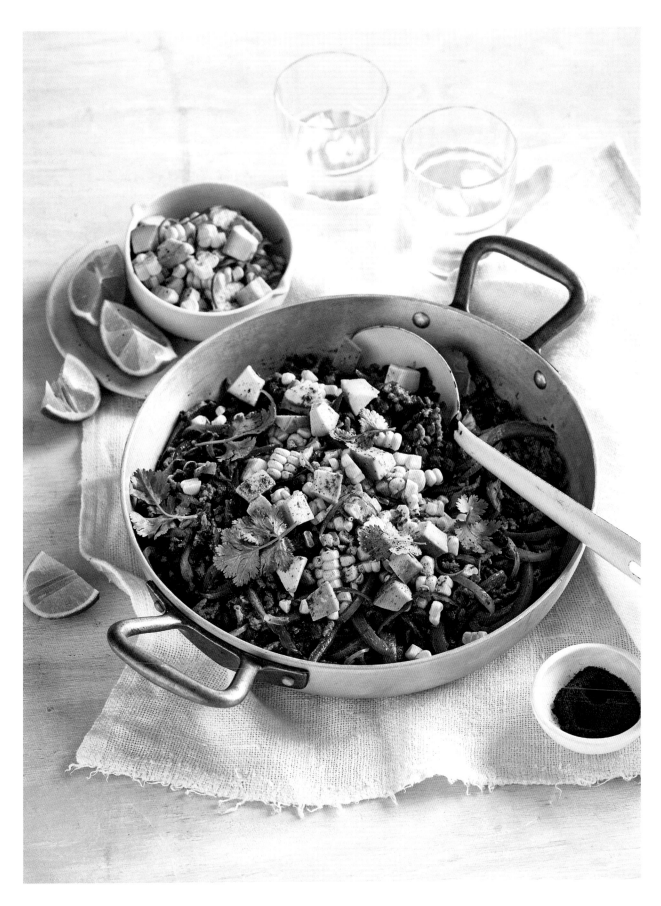

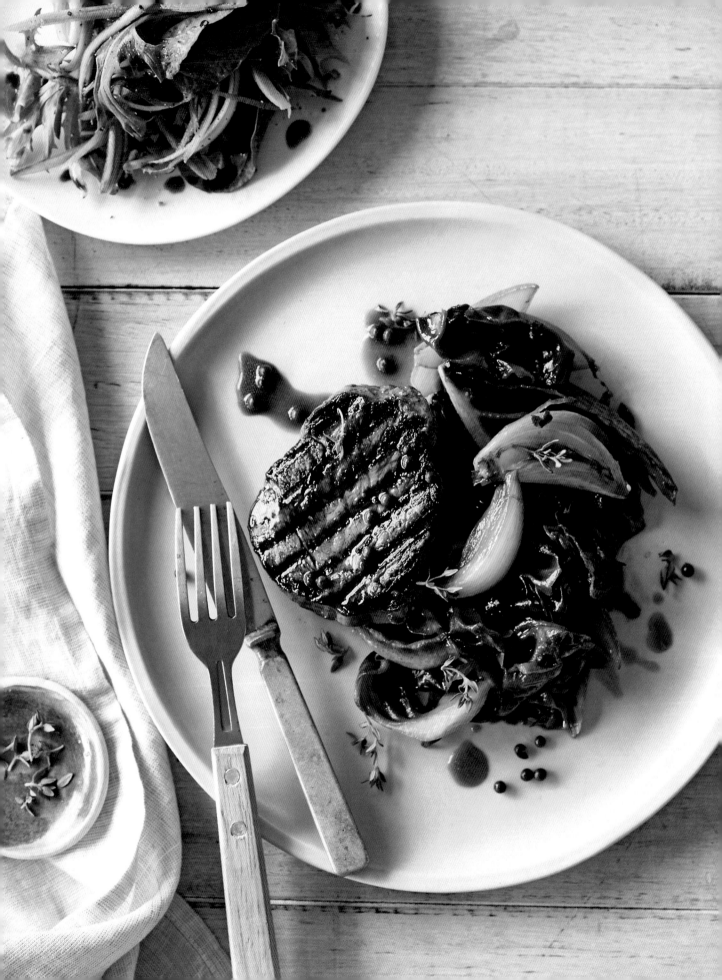

Steak with green peppercorn sauce

Preparation: 20 minutes ✳ **Cooking:** 10 minutes
Difficulty: Easy

SERVES 4

2 teaspoons olive oil

1 tablespoon light margarine

600 g red cabbage, cut into wedges

1 onion, sliced into wedges

1 tablespoon tinned green peppercorns
    in brine, drained (see page 151)

1 cup (250 ml) salt-reduced beef stock

4 x 150 g lean beef fillet steaks

2 cups (60 g) mixed salad leaves

1 Lebanese cucumber, peeled
    into long thin ribbons

1 carrot, peeled into long thin ribbons

1 tablespoon balsamic vinegar

thyme sprigs, to garnish

Heat the olive oil and margarine in a large deep frying pan over medium–high heat. Add the cabbage and onion and cook, turning occasionally, for 5 minutes or until tender and golden. Add the peppercorns and stock and cook, shaking the pan occasionally, for 5 minutes or until the sauce has reduced by half.

Meanwhile, heat a chargrill pan over high heat. Add the steak and cook for 3 minutes each side. Transfer to serving plates and cover loosely with foil to rest and keep warm.

Combine the salad leaves, cucumber, carrot and balsamic in a bowl and season with freshly ground black pepper.

Add the cabbage and peppercorn sauce to the plates with the beef and serve warm garnished with thyme sprigs. Serve the salad alongside.

UNITS PER SERVE Grains **0** ✳ Meat and alternatives **1.5** ✳ Fruit **0** ✳ Vegetables **3.5** ✳ Dairy **0** ✳ Fats and oils **1**

Loaded beef burgers

Preparation: 25 minutes ✳ **Cooking:** 10 minutes
Difficulty: Easy

SERVES 4

400 g lean minced beef

2 teaspoons dried mixed herbs

4 large field mushrooms

light olive oil spray, for cooking

4 large eggs

1 beetroot (about 150 g), peeled
and coarsely grated

1 carrot, coarsely grated

2 spring onions, white and green
parts thinly sliced

2 tablespoons wholegrain mustard

2 tablespoons salt-reduced
barbecue sauce

2 ripe tomatoes, sliced

80 g avocado, sliced

Preheat a barbecue chargrill plate and flat plate to medium–high. Place the minced beef and dried herbs in a bowl and mix with clean hands until well combined. Roll the mixture firmly into four even-sized patties.

Add the patties to the chargrill plate and cook for 5 minutes, then flip them over. Add the mushrooms, cup-side up, to the chargrill plate. Lightly spray the flat plate with olive oil and crack the eggs onto the plate. Cook everything for a further 5 minutes or until the patties and mushrooms are cooked, and the egg whites have set but the yolks are still runny.

Meanwhile, combine the beetroot, carrot, spring onion and mustard in a bowl. Season with freshly ground black pepper.

Transfer the mushrooms to serving plates and spread with the barbecue sauce. Top with the tomato, avocado, patties, eggs and finally the beetroot mixture. Serve hot.

 MAKE IT VEGETARIAN

Replace the beef mince with four vegetarian patties (look for those that contain 14 g of protein or more per patty).

UNITS PER SERVE Grains **0** ✳ Meat and alternatives **1.5** ✳ Fruit **0** ✳ Vegetables **3** ✳ Dairy **0** ✳ Fats and oils **1**

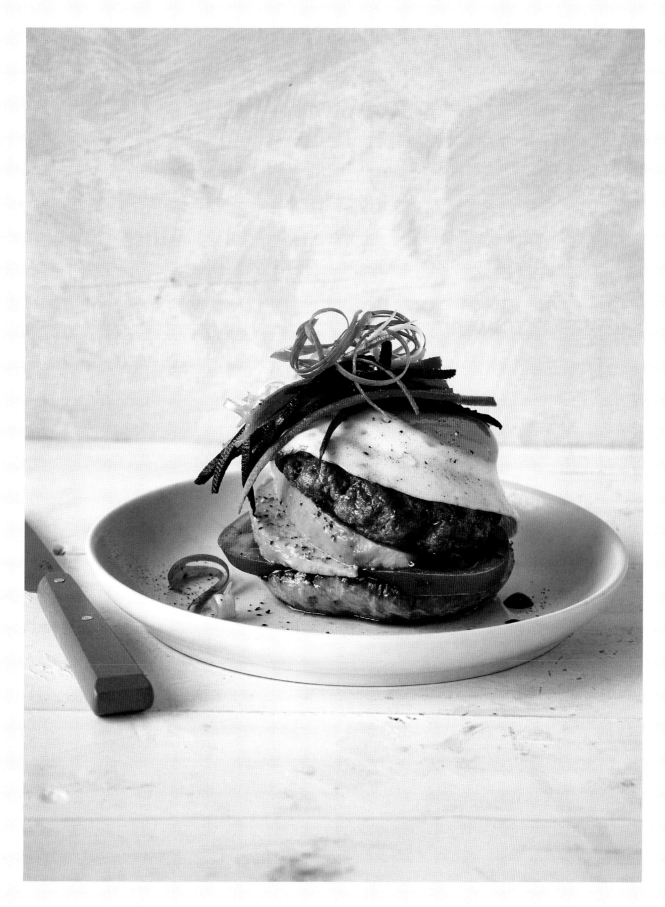

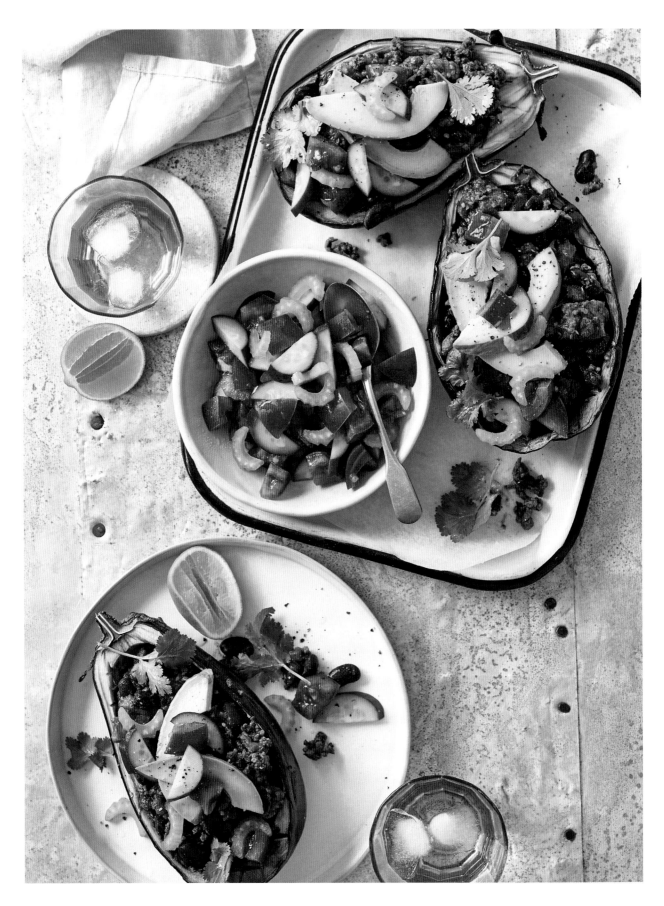

Eggplant Mexicana

Preparation: 15 minutes ✳ **Cooking:** 20 minutes
Difficulty: Medium

SERVES 4

2 large eggplants
light olive oil spray, for cooking
400 g lean minced beef
2 tablespoons salt-reduced tomato paste
1 tablespoon Mexican spice mix
300 g drained, rinsed tinned
    red kidney beans
2 large ripe tomatoes, chopped
2 sticks celery, thinly sliced diagonally
2 Lebanese cucumbers,
    halved lengthways and
    thinly sliced
1 cup small coriander sprigs
80 g avocado, sliced
2 limes, cut into wedges

Preheat the oven to 220°C (200°C fan-forced). Line a large baking tray with baking paper.

Cut the eggplants in half lengthways. Score the flesh into small cubes, then scoop it out with a teaspoon and transfer to a large non-stick frying pan. Place the eggplant shells on the prepared tray, lightly spray with olive oil and season with freshly ground black pepper. Bake for 15 minutes.

Meanwhile, heat the frying pan with the eggplant cubes over medium–high heat. Add the minced beef and cook, stirring and breaking up any large lumps with the back of a spoon, for 10 minutes or until cooked and golden. Add the tomato paste and spice mix and cook, stirring, for 1 minute or until fragrant. Add the kidney beans and 1 cup (250 ml) water. Reduce the heat to low–medium and cook, stirring occasionally, for 6–8 minutes or until the sauce has reduced slightly and the eggplant is soft.

Combine the tomato, celery, cucumber and coriander in a bowl. Season with freshly ground black pepper.

Spoon the beef mixture evenly into the eggplant shells, then transfer to serving plates. Top with avocado slices, then spoon over the tomato mixture. Serve hot with lime wedges.

NOTES

You will need two 400 g tins of red kidney beans for this recipe. Store any leftover beans in an airtight container in the fridge for up to 3 days or in the freezer for up to 3 months.

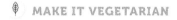

🌿 MAKE IT VEGETARIAN

Replace the beef mince with vegetarian mince.

UNITS PER SERVE Grains **0** ✳ Meat and alternatives **1.5** ✳ Fruit **0** ✳ Vegetables **5** ✳ Dairy **0** ✳ Fats and oils **1**

MAKE IT THREE WAYS

Save time and money, and reduce food waste, by cooking once and turning it into three complete meals.

Beef and lentil braise

Preparation: 25 minutes ✴ **Cooking:** 1 hour 20 minutes
Difficulty: Easy

SERVES 4, WITH LEFTOVERS

light olive oil spray, for cooking
1.2 kg lean beef stir-fry strips
4 onions, chopped
4 sticks celery, chopped
4 large carrots, chopped
8 cloves garlic, sliced
½ cup rosemary leaves
900 g drained, rinsed tinned lentils
  (see Notes)
3 litres salt-reduced beef stock
4 cups (120 g) baby spinach leaves
½ cup small basil leaves
28 g toasted flaked almonds
300 g steamed green beans

Heat a very large saucepan or stockpot over high heat and lightly spray with olive oil. Add one-quarter of the beef strips and cook, stirring, for 2–3 minutes or until browned. Transfer to a bowl. Lightly spray the pan again and, working in three more batches, repeat with the remaining beef.

Lightly spray the pan with olive oil and reduce the heat to medium. Add the onion, celery and carrot and cook, stirring occasionally, for 15 minutes. Return all the meat and any juices to the pan. Add the garlic, rosemary, lentils and stock. Simmer, partially covered, for 45 minutes or until the meat is tender and the sauce has reduced by two-thirds (stirring every now and then). Remove two-thirds of the braise and divide evenly between two airtight containers. Allow to cool before storing (see Notes).

Remove the pan from the heat and add the spinach to the remaining braise mixture, stirring until wilted. Spoon into serving bowls and top with the basil leaves and almonds. Serve with steamed green beans alongside.

NOTES

You will need five 400 g tins of lentils for this recipe. Store any leftover lentils in an airtight container in the fridge for up to 3 days or in the freezer for up to 3 months. Leftover braise can be stored in airtight containers in the fridge for up to 2 days or in the freezer for up to 3 months. Thaw the frozen mixture in the fridge overnight. Reheat in a large saucepan over medium heat for 15–20 minutes or until hot.

UNITS PER SERVE Grains **0** ✴ Meat and alternatives **1.5**
Fruit **0** ✴ Vegetables **3** ✴ Dairy **0** ✴ Fats and oils **1**

USING THE LEFTOVERS...

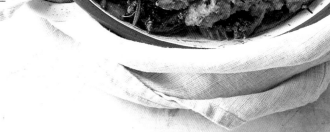

Mexican chilli

Preparation: 15 minutes ✳ **Cooking:** 15 minutes
Difficulty: Easy

SERVES 4

Place one portion of the leftovers in a large saucepan and add 2 tablespoons tomato paste and 1 x 30 g packet salt-reduced taco spice blend. Cook over medium heat, stirring occasionally, for 15 minutes or until heated through. Divide among four bowls and top with 80 g sliced avocado, ½ cup coriander leaves and 2 sliced spring onions. Serve with lime wedges alongside.

UNITS PER SERVE Grains **0** ✳ Meat and alternatives **1.5** ✳ Fruit **0** ✳ Vegetables **3** ✳ Dairy **0** ✳ Fats and oils **1**

Beef and lentil bake

Preparation: 15 minutes ✳ **Cooking:** 20 minutes
Difficulty: Easy

SERVES 4

Preheat the oven grill to high. Place 2 cups (200 g) cauliflower florets and 500 g peeled, seeded and chopped pumpkin in a saucepan of water and boil for 12–15 minutes or until tender. Drain and return to the pan, then mash with 2 tablespoons light margarine. Meanwhile, place one portion of the leftovers in a large saucepan and heat over medium heat for 10 minutes or until hot. Spoon into a 1.5 litre flameproof baking dish and top with the mash. Place under the grill for 3–5 minutes or until golden and crisp. Serve hot with mixed salad greens.

UNITS PER SERVE Grains **0** ✳ Meat and alternatives **1.5** ✳ Fruit **0** ✳ Vegetables **5** ✳ Dairy **0** ✳ Fats and oils **1**

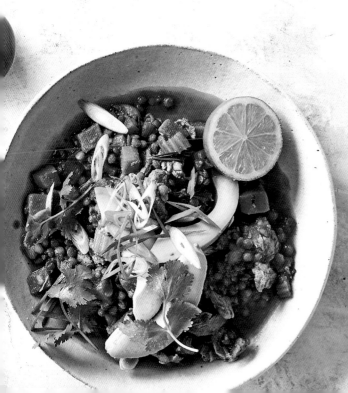

Harissa lamb and chickpea roast

Preparation: 15 minutes, plus resting time ✳ **Cooking:** 35 minutes
Difficulty: Easy

SERVES 4

2 x 400 g tins cherry tomatoes
2 spring onions, white and
    green parts sliced
300 g drained, rinsed tinned chickpeas
2 zucchini, chopped into 2 cm dice
300 g peeled, seeded butternut
    pumpkin, chopped into 2 cm dice
1 cup (250 ml) salt-reduced beef stock
1 tablespoon olive oil
2 tablespoons harissa spice seasoning
400 g lean lamb mini roast
1 cup (120 g) frozen baby peas, thawed
basil leaves, to serve

Preheat the oven to 200°C (180°C fan-forced).

Combine the tomatoes, spring onion, chickpeas, zucchini, pumpkin and stock in a heavy-based baking dish and bake for 15 minutes.

Meanwhile, place the olive oil and seasoning in a bowl, add the lamb and toss to coat well on all sides.

Add the lamb to the baking dish, scraping over any leftover spiced oil from the bowl. Bake for 20 minutes for medium or until cooked to your liking. Remove from the oven and add the peas to the dish. Cover loosely with foil and leave to rest for 5 minutes before removing and slicing the lamb.

Return the sliced lamb to the chickpea mixture, then take the dish to the table. Garnish with basil leaves before serving.

NOTES

You will need two 400 g tins of chickpeas for this recipe. Store any leftover chickpeas in an airtight container in the fridge for up to 3 days or in the freezer for up to 3 months.

UNITS PER SERVE Grains **0** ✳ Meat and alternatives **1.5** ✳ Fruit **0** ✳ Vegetables **5** ✳ Dairy **0** ✳ Fats and oils **1**

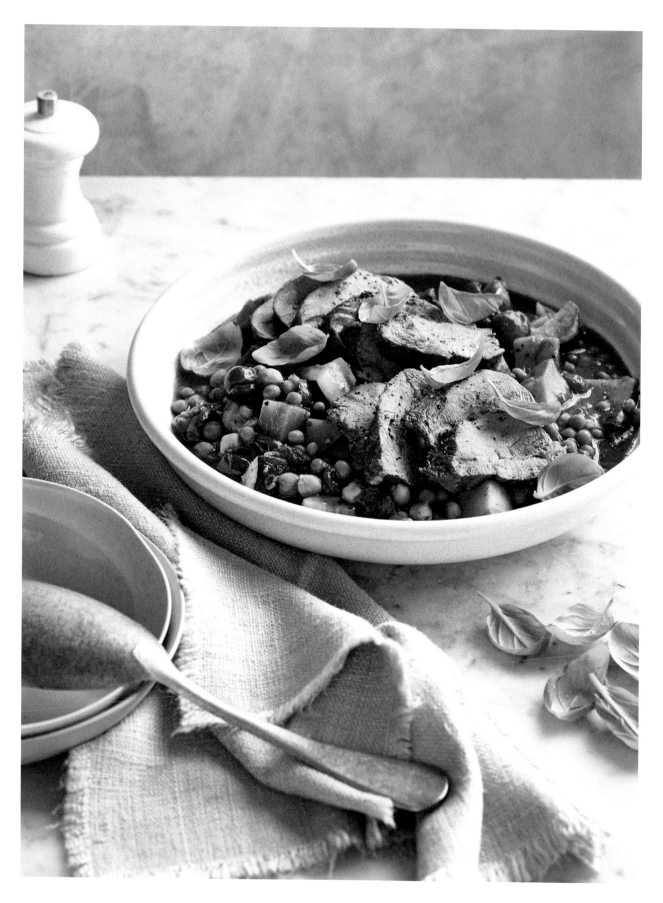

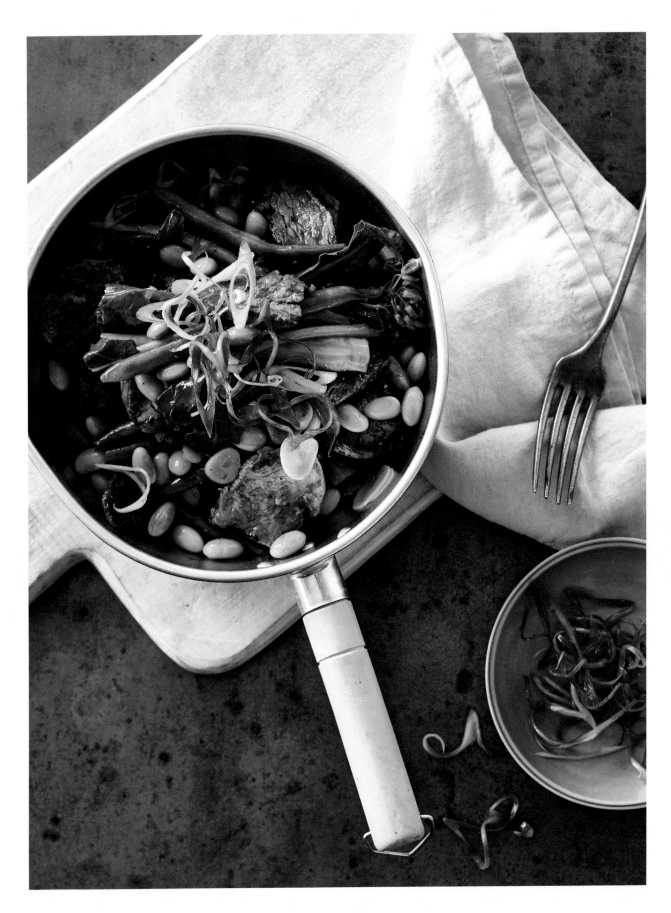

Sticky pork and garlic greens

Preparation: 15 minutes, plus chilling time ✳ **Cooking:** 10 minutes
Difficulty: Easy

SERVES 4

2 tablespoons salt-reduced hoisin sauce

2 tablespoons salt-reduced oyster sauce

2 tablespoons salt-reduced tomato sauce

600 g lean pork fillet, sinew
    removed, cut into 1 cm thick slices

1 tablespoon sunflower oil

1 bunch Chinese broccoli,
    trimmed and halved

300 g green beans, trimmed

4 cloves garlic, thinly sliced

300 g frozen shelled edamame, thawed

finely sliced spring onion, to serve

Combine the sauces and pork in a large non-metallic bowl and season with freshly ground black pepper. Cover and chill for at least 1 hour, or overnight if time permits.

Heat half the sunflower oil in a large non-stick wok over high heat. Add the pork mixture and stir-fry for 5 minutes or until cooked and dark golden. Transfer to a heatproof bowl and cover to keep warm.

Heat the remaining oil in the wok, add the Chinese broccoli, beans and garlic and stir-fry for 1 minute. Add the edamame and ⅓ cup (80 ml) water and stir-fry for 1 minute. Return the pork and any juices to the wok and toss well, then remove from the heat. Spoon the pork and greens into bowls and serve garnished with spring onion.

UNITS PER SERVE Grains **0** ✳ Meat and alternatives **1.5** ✳ Fruit **0** ✳ Vegetables **3** ✳ Dairy **0** ✳ Fats and oils **1**

Pork and pistachio loaf

Preparation: 25 minutes, plus resting time ✳ **Cooking:** 50 minutes
Difficulty: Easy

SERVES 4

550 g lean minced pork fillet
1 large egg
2 large spring onions, white and
    green parts thinly sliced
1 carrot, coarsely grated
1 stick celery, finely chopped
2 tablespoons salt-reduced
    barbecue sauce
2 tablespoons finely chopped
    flat-leaf parsley
28 g unsalted shelled pistachios,
    finely chopped
½ teaspoon freshly ground black pepper
2 teaspoons fennel seeds (optional)
light olive oil spray, for cooking
3 cups (255 g) broccoli florets
2 tablespoons apple cider vinegar
250 g grape tomatoes, halved lengthways
1 cup (30 g) baby rocket leaves

Preheat the oven to 200°C (180°C fan-forced). Line the base and sides of a 20 cm x 10 cm loaf tin with baking paper.

Combine the pork, egg, spring onion, carrot, celery, barbecue sauce and parsley in a large bowl and mix with clean hands until no air bubbles are left and the pork feels sticky. Press the mixture firmly into the prepared tin and sprinkle evenly with the combined pistachio, pepper and fennel seeds (if using). Lightly spray the top with olive oil.

Bake for 50 minutes or until golden and cooked when tested in the centre with a skewer. Rest in the tin for 5 minutes before removing and slicing.

Meanwhile, heat a chargrill pan over high heat. Lightly spray the broccoli with olive oil and chargrill for 2–3 minutes or until just tender. Transfer to a large bowl and add the vinegar, tomatoes and rocket. Toss to combine well and season with freshly ground black pepper.

Serve the sliced pork loaf with the broccoli salad.

NOTES

This loaf is delicious hot or cold so it's a good one to make ahead of time. Store in an airtight container in the fridge for up to 2 days or in the freezer for 3 months. Bring it to room temperature or gently warm through to serve.

UNITS PER SERVE
Grains **0** ✳ Meat and alternatives **1.5**
Fruit **0** ✳ Vegetables **3** ✳ Dairy **0**
Fats and oils **1**

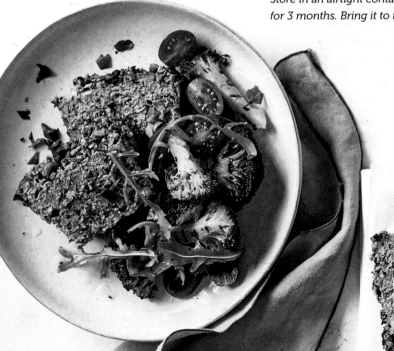
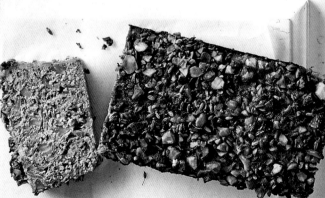

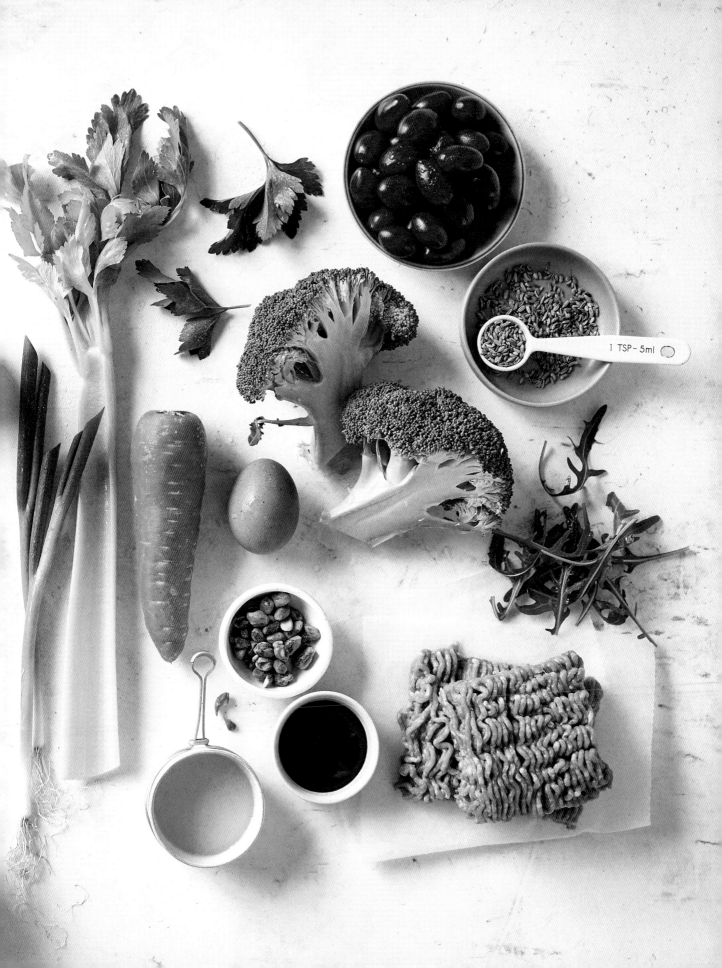

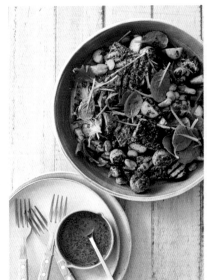

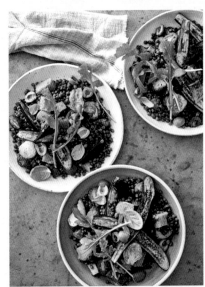

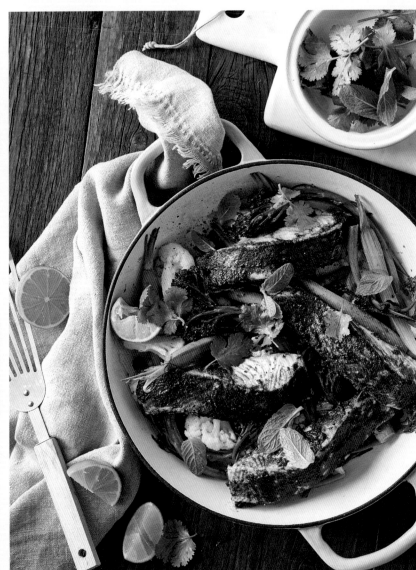

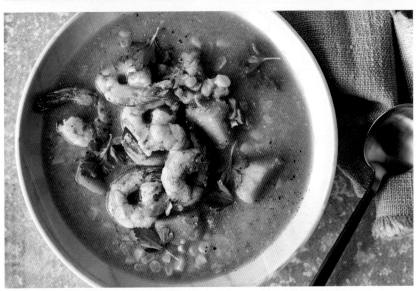

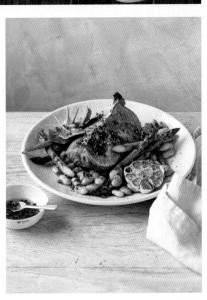

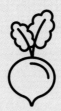

5. Seafood and Vegetarian Dinners

Grilled fish with ginger oil

Preparation: 20 minutes ✶ **Cooking:** 15 minutes
Difficulty: Medium

SERVES 4

light olive oil spray, for cooking
600 g firm white fish fillets,
    skin removed and pin-boned
2 bunches asparagus, trimmed
350 g sugar snap peas, trimmed
350 g snowpeas, trimmed
2 tablespoons salt-reduced soy sauce
2 spring onions, white and green
    parts thinly sliced

GINGER OIL
1 tablespoon sunflower oil
1 tablespoon finely chopped ginger
1 clove garlic, crushed

Preheat the oven grill to high. Lightly spray a large non-stick baking tray with a 1 cm lip with olive oil.

Add the fish to the prepared tray, then add the asparagus, sugar snaps and snowpeas. Lightly spray with olive oil and season with freshly ground black pepper. Cook under the grill, turning the vegetables once, for 10–12 minutes or until the fish is cooked and lightly golden. (Don't turn the fish – it's too delicate and will break.) Remove the tray from the grill and sprinkle the soy sauce and spring onion over the fish.

Shortly before the fish is ready, make the ginger oil. Heat the sunflower oil in a small saucepan over medium heat until almost smoking. Remove the pan from the heat and add the ginger and garlic straight away, shaking gently to combine. Immediately pour evenly over the hot fish and serve.

UNITS PER SERVE Grains **0** ✶ Meat and alternatives **1.5** ✶ Fruit **0** ✶ Vegetables **3** ✶ Dairy **0** ✶ Fats and oils **1**

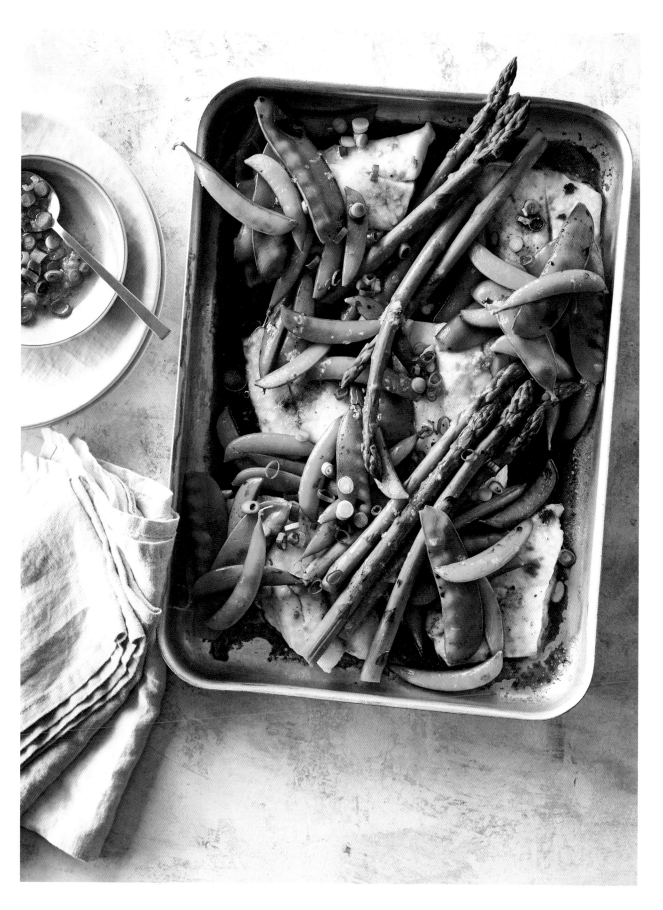

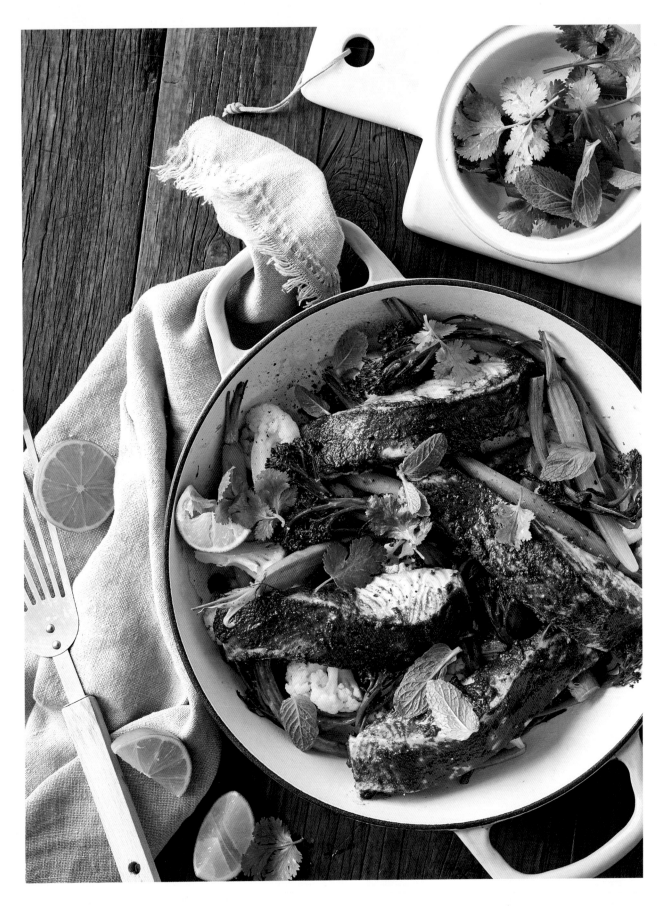

Tandoori salmon

Preparation: 15 minutes, plus chilling time ✳ **Cooking:** 20 minutes
Difficulty: Easy

SERVES 4

¼ cup (75 g) tandoori curry paste

4 x 150 g salmon fillets, skin removed and pin-boned

2 cups (200 g) cauliflower florets

1 bunch baby carrots, trimmed, scrubbed, halved lengthways

½ cup (125 ml) salt-reduced chicken stock

1 bunch broccolini, trimmed and halved lengthways

light olive oil spray, for cooking

½ cup small mint leaves

½ cup small coriander sprigs

lime wedges, to serve

Using clean hands, rub the curry paste over the salmon, covering all sides evenly. Cover and chill for at least 20 minutes to marinate.

Preheat the oven grill to high.

Combine the cauliflower, carrots and stock in a large, deep flameproof frying pan over medium–high heat. Bring to the boil and cook, stirring occasionally, for 5 minutes. Add the broccolini and cook for a further 3 minutes or until all the vegetables are tender.

Rest the salmon on top of the vegetables and lightly spray with olive oil. Cook under the grill for 10 minutes or until the salmon is just cooked and golden. Remove the pan from the grill and sprinkle over the mint and coriander. Take the pan to the table and serve with lime wedges.

UNITS PER SERVE Grains **0** ✳ Meat and alternatives **1.5** ✳ Fruit **0** ✳ Vegetables **3.5** ✳ Dairy **0** ✳ Fats and oils **1**

Prawn, pumpkin and corn chowder

Preparation: 20 minutes ✳ **Cooking:** 25 minutes
Difficulty: Easy

SERVES 4

2 tablespoons light margarine
600 g peeled and deveined raw
    medium king prawns, tails intact
1 onion, finely chopped
2 cloves garlic, crushed
500 g peeled, seeded butternut
    pumpkin, chopped
4 cobs sweetcorn, husks and silks
    removed, kernels sliced off
1.5 litres salt-reduced chicken stock
2 tablespoons chopped
    flat-leaf parsley

Melt half the margarine in a large heavy-based saucepan over medium–high heat. Add the prawns and cook, tossing, for 4–5 minutes or until cooked through. Transfer to a heatproof bowl and season with freshly ground black pepper, then cover to keep warm.

Reduce the heat to medium. Melt the remaining margarine in the pan, then add the onion and garlic and cook, stirring, for 3 minutes. Add the pumpkin, corn and stock and cook, stirring occasionally, for 15 minutes or until the pumpkin is tender.

Transfer half the mixture to an upright blender and blend until smooth, then return to the pan. Stir well to combine and season with freshly ground black pepper.

Divide the chowder among serving bowls and top with the prawns and any juices. Sprinkle with parsley and serve.

UNITS PER SERVE Grains **0** ✳ Meat and alternatives **1.5** ✳ Fruit **0** ✳ Vegetables **3.5** ✳ Dairy **0** ✳ Fats and oils **1**

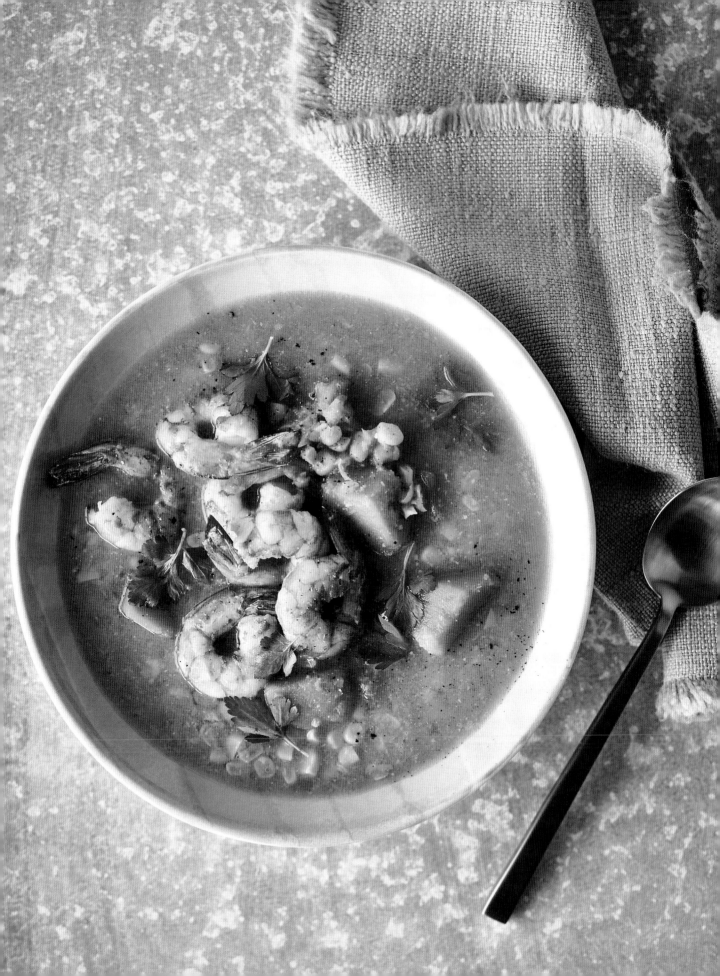

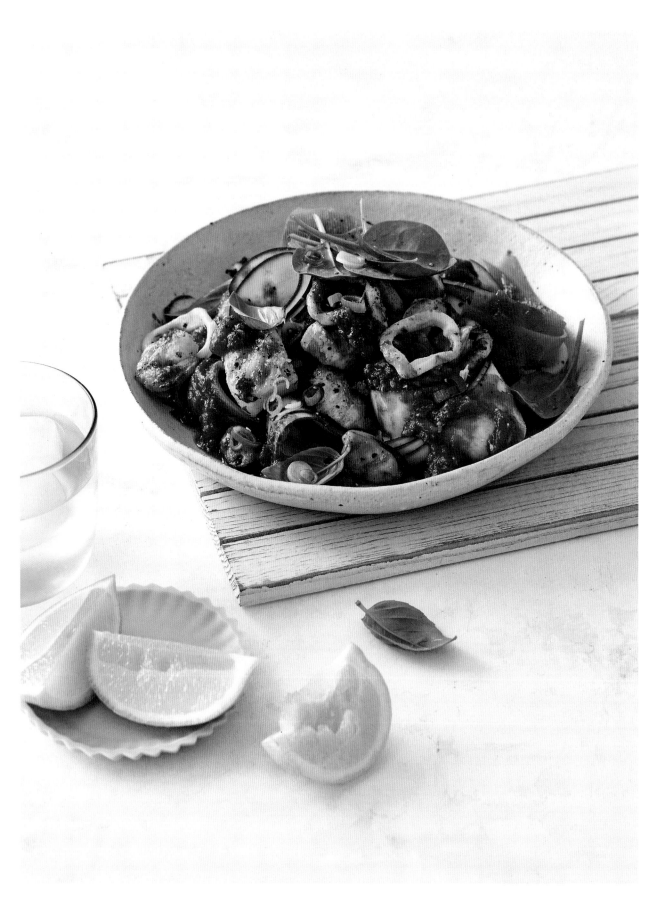

Chargrilled marinara on vegetable pappardelle

Preparation: 20 minutes * **Cooking:** 10 minutes
Difficulty: Easy

SERVES 4

1 tablespoon olive oil
2 cloves garlic, crushed
2 x 400 g tins whole peeled tomatoes
1 cup basil leaves
600 g fresh marinara mix
4 carrots, cut into long thin ribbons
    using a vegetable peeler
4 zucchini, cut into long thin ribbons
    using a vegetable peeler
1 cup (30 g) baby spinach leaves
2 spring onions, white and green
    parts thinly sliced
lemon wedges, to serve

Preheat a large chargrill pan over high heat.

Heat the olive oil in a large deep frying pan over medium–high heat. Add the garlic, tomatoes and basil and cook, stirring and crushing the tomatoes, for 10 minutes or until reduced by half.

Meanwhile, add half the marinara mix to the chargrill pan and cook for 5 minutes or until the seafood is just cooked and golden. Transfer to a heatproof bowl and repeat with the remaining seafood. Season with freshly ground black pepper and cover to keep warm.

Add the carrot, zucchini and baby spinach to the tomato mixture and toss very gently to combine and coat well. Immediately remove from the heat and divide among serving bowls. Top with the seafood and any juices, sprinkle with the spring onion and serve with wedges of lemon.

UNITS PER SERVE Grains **0** * Meat and alternatives **1.5** * Fruit **0** * Vegetables **6** * Dairy **0** * Fats and oils **1**

Korma chickpeas and cabbage

Preparation: 15 minutes ✳ **Cooking:** 20 minutes
Difficulty: Easy

SERVES 4

¼ cup (75 g) korma curry paste
1 tablespoon garam masala
1 tablespoon finely chopped ginger
1 onion, thinly sliced
900 g drained, rinsed tinned chickpeas
500 g red cabbage, cut into 4 cm chunks
1 litre salt-reduced vegetable stock
3 zucchini, diced
¼ cup small flat-leaf parsley leaves

Heat the curry paste in a large deep frying pan over medium heat. Add the garam masala, ginger and onion and cook, stirring occasionally, for 3 minutes or until just starting to soften.

Add the chickpeas, cabbage and stock and cook, stirring occasionally, for 10 minutes. Add the zucchini and cook, stirring occasionally, for 3 minutes or until just tender. Sprinkle with parsley and serve.

NOTES

You will need five 400 g tins of chickpeas for this recipe. Leftover chickpeas can be stored in an airtight container in the fridge for up to 3 days or in the freezer for up to 3 months.

UNITS PER SERVE Grains **0** ✳ Meat and alternatives **2** ✳ Fruit **0** ✳ Vegetables **3** ✳ Dairy **0** ✳ Fats and oils **1**

Egg green curry

Preparation: 20 minutes ✳ **Cooking:** 10 minutes
Difficulty: Medium

SERVES 4

8 large eggs

3 tablespoons Thai green curry paste

4 spring onions, white and green parts
  cut into 4 cm lengths

2 zucchini, cut into thick matchsticks

200 g green beans, trimmed

2 cups (170 g) broccoli florets

300 g frozen shelled edamame, thawed

1 cup (250 ml) salt-reduced
  vegetable stock

1 tablespoon salt-reduced soy sauce

1 cup (80 g) bean sprouts, trimmed

½ cup coriander leaves

Cook the eggs in a large saucepan of boiling water for 6 minutes. Drain, then carefully remove the shells under cold running water. Cut the eggs in half lengthways and set aside.

Heat the curry paste in a large wok over high heat. Add the spring onion, zucchini, beans, broccoli, edamame, stock and soy sauce and stir-fry for 3 minutes or until the vegetables are just tender and the sauce has reduced slightly.

Divide the vegetable mixture among serving bowls. Top with the boiled eggs, bean sprouts and coriander, and serve.

UNITS PER SERVE Grains **0** ✳ Meat and alternatives **1.5** ✳ Fruit **0** ✳ Vegetables **3** ✳ Dairy **0** ✳ Fats and oils **1**

Paprika tofu and chimichurri vegetables

Preparation: 20 minutes ✽ **Cooking:** 10 minutes
Difficulty: Easy

SERVES 4

680 g firm tofu, sliced

2 tablespoons smoked paprika

500 g button mushrooms

light olive oil spray, for cooking

300 g frozen shelled broad beans,
    thawed and peeled

4 cups (120 g) baby leaves and
    beetroot salad mix (see Notes)

2 Lebanese cucumbers, sliced

CHIMICHURRI

½ cup flat-leaf parsley leaves

½ cup coriander leaves

¼ cup oregano leaves

⅓ cup (80 ml) red wine vinegar

1 tablespoon extra virgin olive oil

1 clove garlic, roughly chopped

To make the chimichurri, place all the ingredients in a small food processor and blend until smooth. Season with freshly ground black pepper, then transfer to a large heatproof bowl.

Preheat a large chargrill pan over high heat. Toss the tofu in the paprika, coating it evenly on all sides. Lightly spray the tofu and mushrooms with olive oil. Working in two batches, add to the chargrill pan and cook, turning occasionally, for 5 minutes or until cooked and golden. Add to the chimichurri in the bowl and toss well to combine.

Add the broad beans, salad mix and cucumber to the tofu mixture and gently toss to combine. Serve warm.

NOTES

You can buy prepacked baby leaves and beetroot salad mix at large supermarkets.

UNITS PER SERVE Grains **0** ✽ Meat and alternatives **1.5** ✽ Fruit **0** ✽ Vegetables **3** ✽ Dairy **0** ✽ Fats and oils **1**

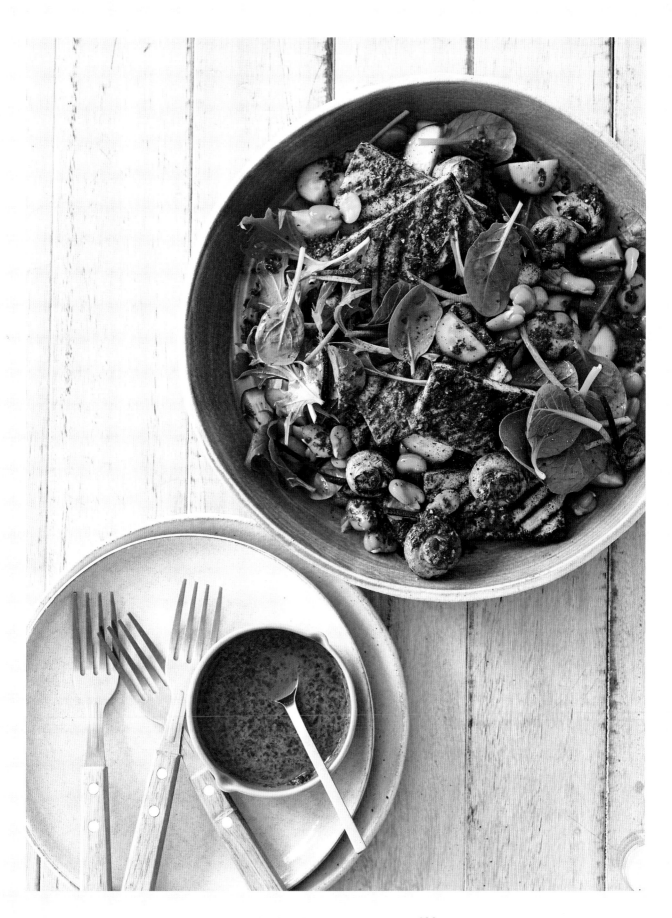

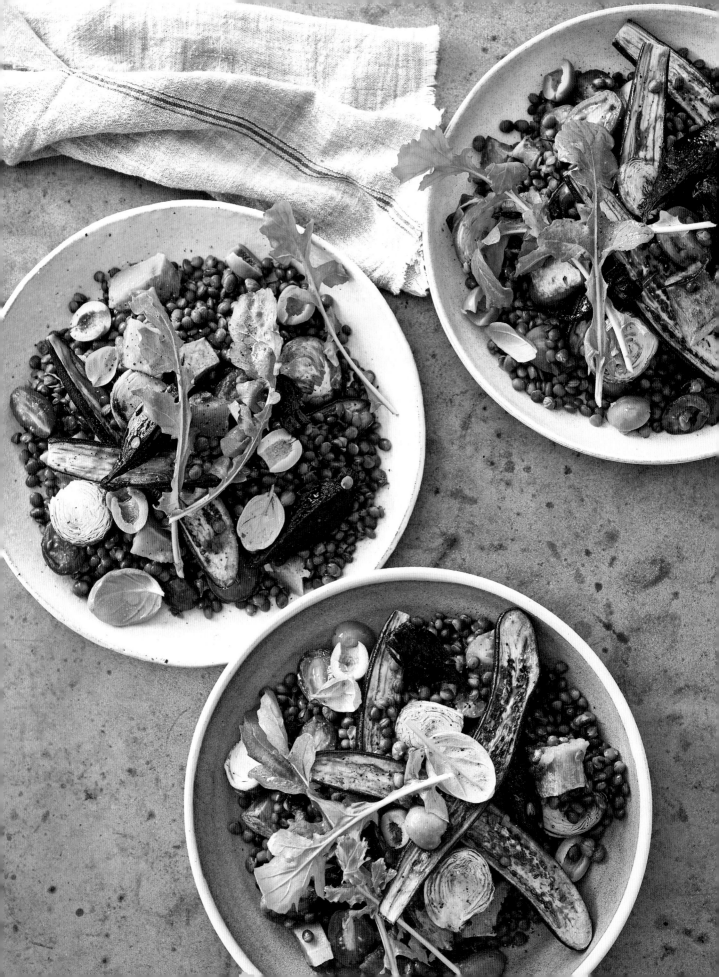

Italian vegetable roast

Preparation: 20 minutes ✳ **Cooking:** 45 minutes
Difficulty: Medium

SERVES 4

1 bunch baby beetroot, trimmed
   and quartered
500 g peeled, seeded butternut pumpkin,
   cut into 3 cm pieces
1 tablespoon garlic-infused olive oil
¼ cup rosemary leaves
8 baby eggplants, halved lengthways
500 g Brussels sprouts, trimmed
   and halved
500 g mixed cherry tomatoes, halved
900 g drained, rinsed tinned lentils
2 tablespoons baby capers
   in brine, rinsed
½ cup (60 g) pitted green olives, halved
1 cup small basil leaves
handful of baby rocket and
   spinach leaves, to serve

Preheat the oven to 200°C (180°C fan-forced).

Combine the beetroot, pumpkin, olive oil and rosemary in a heavy-based baking dish. Bake for 20 minutes. Add the eggplant and sprouts and toss to combine, then bake for a further 15 minutes.

Add the tomatoes, lentils and ½ cup (125 ml) water and toss well to combine. Bake for 10 minutes. Remove the dish from the oven and immediately add the capers, olives and basil. Toss together well and season with freshly ground black pepper.

Divide the vegetable mixture among bowls, scatter over the rocket and spinach leaves and serve hot.

NOTES

You will need five 400 g tins of lentils for this recipe. Leftover lentils can be stored in an airtight container in the fridge for up to 3 days or in the freezer for up to 3 months.

UNITS PER SERVE Grains **0** ✳ Meat and alternatives **1.5** ✳ Fruit **0** ✳ Vegetables **8** ✳ Dairy **0** ✳ Fats and oils **1**

Roast pumpkin and butter beans

Preparation: 15 minutes ✳ **Cooking:** 1 hour 10 minutes
Difficulty: Easy

SERVES 4

1.25 kg butternut pumpkin, ends
    trimmed, quartered lengthways,
    seeds and skin left on
2 heads garlic, excess papery skin
    removed, halved horizontally
light olive oil spray, for cooking
2 tablespoons fennel seeds
900 g drained, rinsed tinned butter beans
2 bunches asparagus, trimmed and
    thickly sliced diagonally
½ cup baby spinach leaves
1 tablespoon extra virgin olive oil
⅓ cup (80 ml) white wine vinegar
2 tablespoons finely chopped chives

Preheat the oven to 180°C (160°C fan-forced).

Place the pumpkin wedges, skin-side down, side by side in a large heavy-based baking dish. Nestle the garlic, cut side up, around the pumpkin. Lightly spray with olive oil, sprinkle with fennel seeds and season with freshly ground black pepper. Roast for 1 hour or until tender and golden.

Add the butter beans and asparagus to the dish and lightly spray with olive oil. Roast for a further 10 minutes or until the beans are heated through and the asparagus is just tender.

Divide among serving plates and scatter over the baby spinach leaves.

Combine the olive oil, vinegar and chives in a small jug and season with freshly ground black pepper. Pour over the dressing and serve.

NOTE

You will need five 400 g tins of butter beans for this recipe. Leftover beans can be stored in an airtight container in the fridge for up to 3 days or in the freezer for up to 3 months.

UNITS PER SERVE Grains **0** ✳ Meat and alternatives **1.5** ✳ Fruit **0** ✳ Vegetables **4.5** ✳ Dairy **0** ✳ Fats and oils **1**

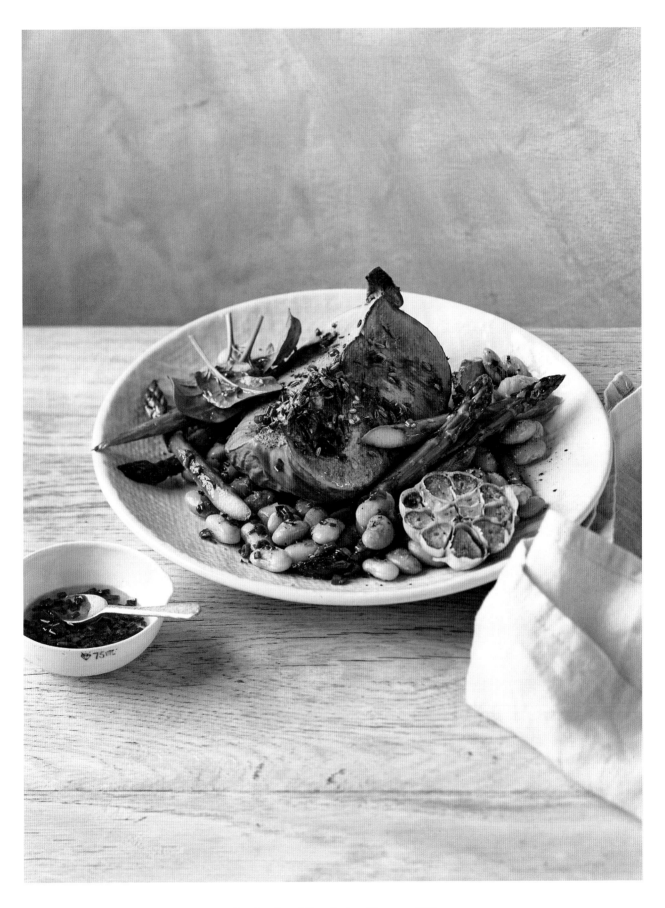

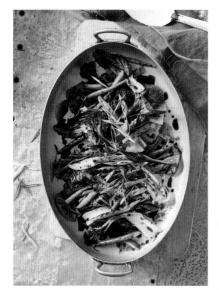

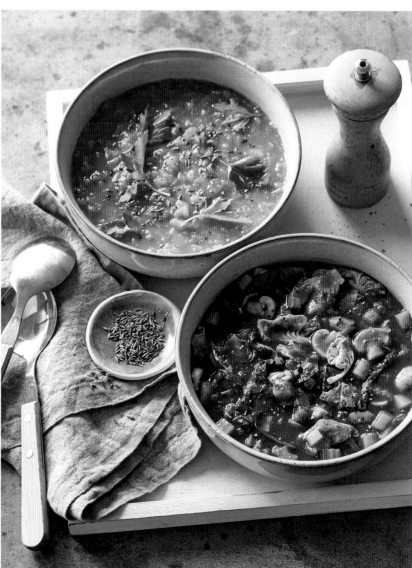

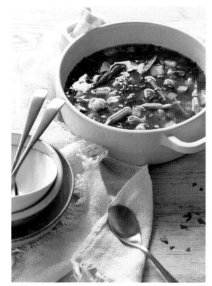

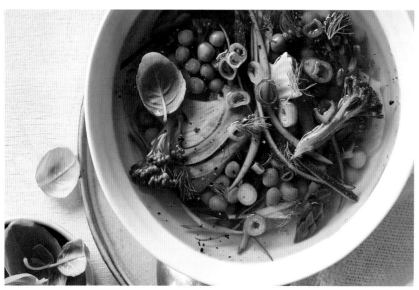

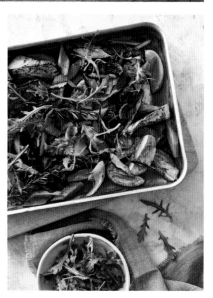

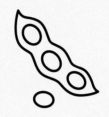

6. Vegetable Sides and Soups

Cauliflower and zucchini 'rice'

Preparation: 15 minutes
Cooking: nil
Difficulty: Easy

2 cups (200 g) cauliflower florets (about ½ cauliflower)
2 zucchini, trimmed and chopped
2 tablespoons finely chopped chives
ground white pepper, to taste

Working in batches, separately process the cauliflower and zucchini in a food processor until finely chopped. Combine in a bowl with the chives and season to taste with white pepper. Serve.

NOTES

If you don't have a food processor you can simply grate the cauliflower and zucchini using the larger holes on a box grater.

You can serve this 'rice' raw or cooked. To cook, place in a large deep frying pan with 2 tablespoons water. Cook, tossing, over medium–high heat for 2–3 minutes or until just tender.

Carrot, swede and cauliflower mash

Preparation: 15 minutes
Cooking: 30 minutes
Difficulty: Easy

SERVES 4

4 carrots, chopped
1 swede (about 300 g), peeled and cut into 1 cm pieces
2 cups (200 g) cauliflower florets
2–3 tablespoons salt-reduced vegetable stock

Cook the carrot and swede in a large saucepan of boiling water over high heat for 20 minutes. Add the cauliflower and boil for a further 10 minutes. Drain well.

Transfer the vegetables to a blender and blend until smooth and creamy, adding just enough stock to loosen. Season with freshly ground black pepper and serve.

UNITS PER SERVE Grains **0** * Meat and alternatives **0**
Fruit **0** * Vegetables **2** * Dairy **0** * Fats and oils **0**

UNITS PER SERVE Grains **0** * Meat and alternatives **0**
* Fruit **0** * Vegetables **3** * Dairy **0** * Fats and oils **0**

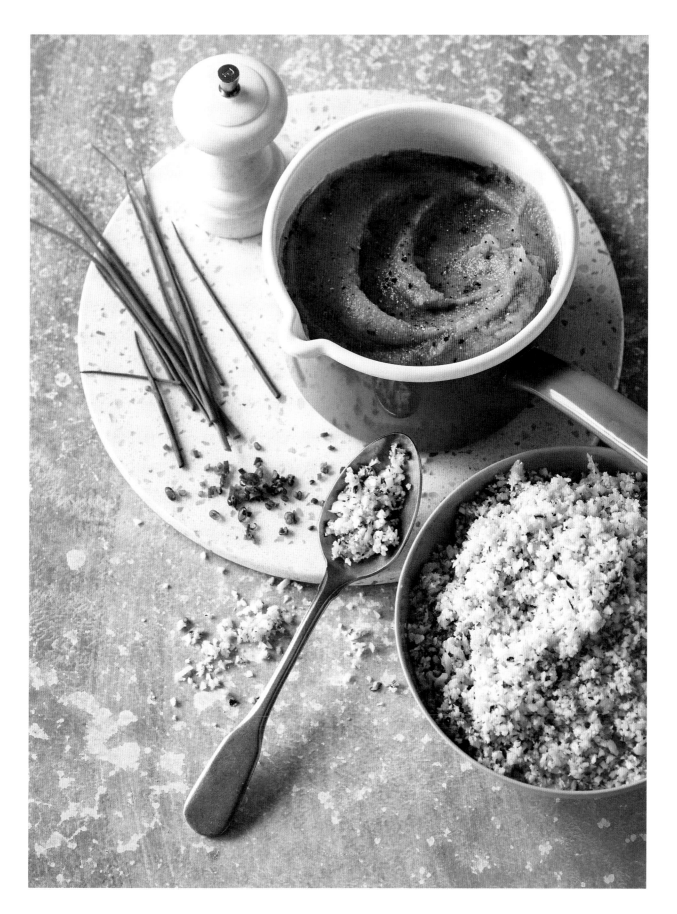

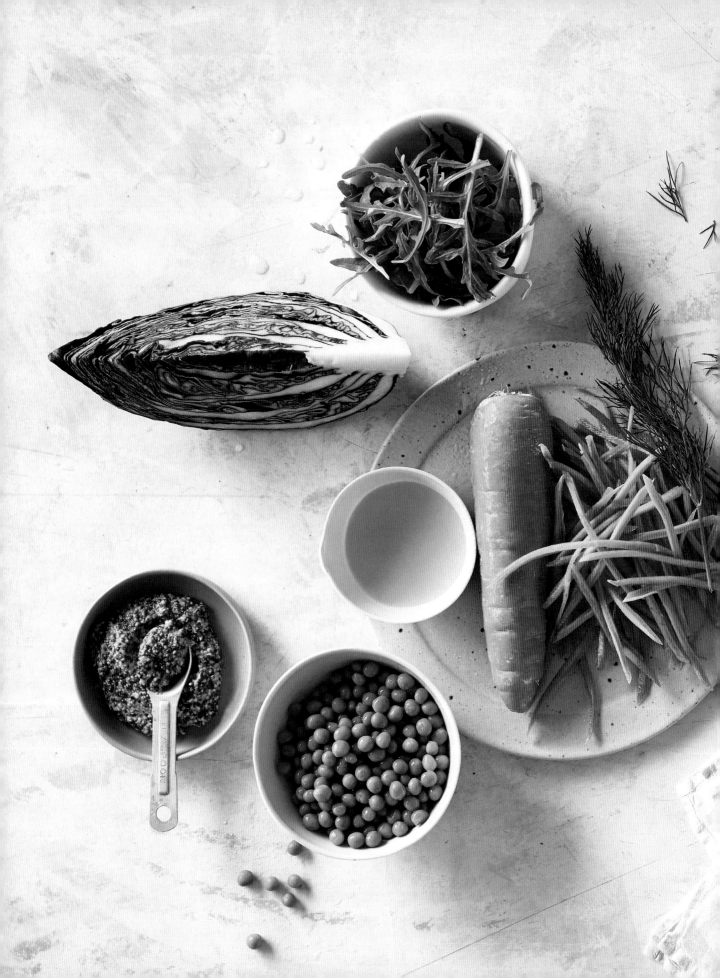

Dill, cabbage and pea slaw

Preparation: 15 minutes ✽ **Cooking:** nil
Difficulty: Easy

SERVES 4

1 cup (120 g) frozen peas, thawed
200 g red cabbage, very thinly sliced
2 carrots, coarsely grated
20 g baby rocket leaves

DILL DRESSING
2 tablespoons dill leaves
¼ cup (60 ml) apple cider vinegar
1 teaspoon wholegrain mustard

To make the dill dressing, combine all the ingredients in a large bowl. Season with freshly ground black pepper.

Add the peas, cabbage, carrot and rocket to the dill dressing and toss well to combine. Serve.

NOTES

If you are short on time you can quickly thaw the peas by placing them in a colander and running cold tap water over them. Using cold water will keep the colour nice and vibrant.

UNITS PER SERVE Grains **0** ✽ Meat and alternatives **0** ✽ Fruit **0** ✽ Vegetables **2** ✽ Dairy **0** ✽ Fats and oils **0**

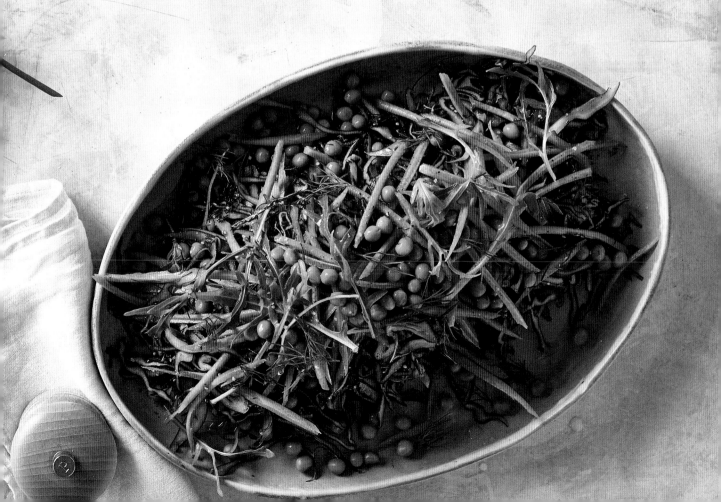

Chargrilled Asian greens

Preparation: 15 minutes ✳ **Cooking:** 10 minutes
Difficulty: Easy

SERVES 4

2 tablespoons salt-reduced soy sauce
1 tablespoon salt-reduced hoisin sauce
2 spring onions, white and green parts
   thinly sliced
1 bunch broccolini, trimmed
   and halved lengthways
200 g green beans, trimmed
1 bunch (3 pieces) baby bok choy,
   halved lengthways

Preheat a barbecue chargrill plate to medium–high.

Combine the soy sauce, hoisin sauce and spring onion in a large heatproof bowl. Season with freshly ground black pepper.

Working in batches, chargrill the broccolini, beans and bok choy, turning occasionally, for 2–3 minutes or until just tender. Immediately transfer the vegetables to the soy sauce mixture and toss well to combine. Serve warm.

UNITS PER SERVE Grains **0** ✳ Meat and alternatives **0** ✳ Fruit **0** ✳ Vegetables **2** ✳ Dairy **0** ✳ Fats and oils **0**

210 CSIRO Protein Plus

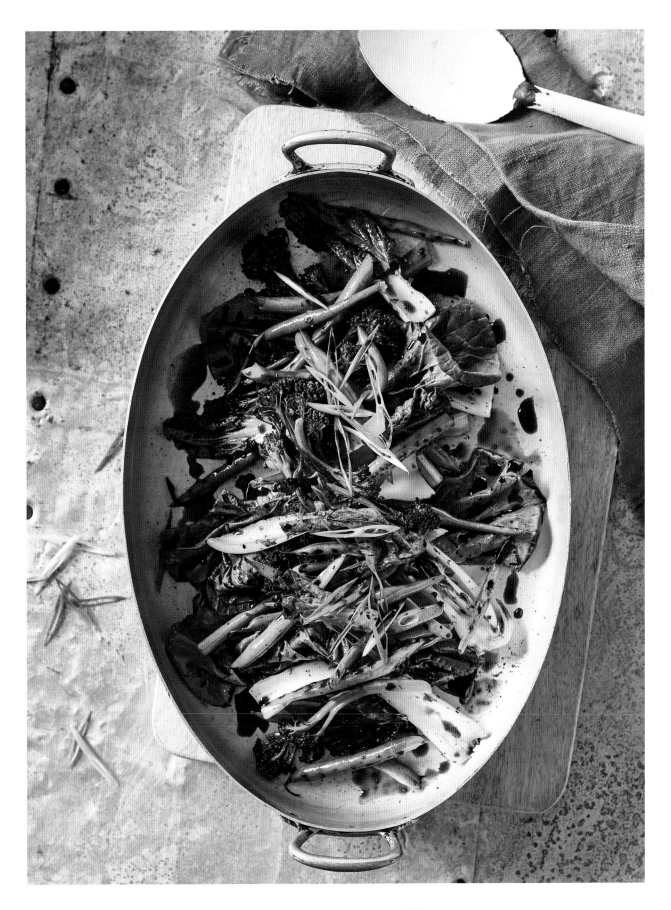

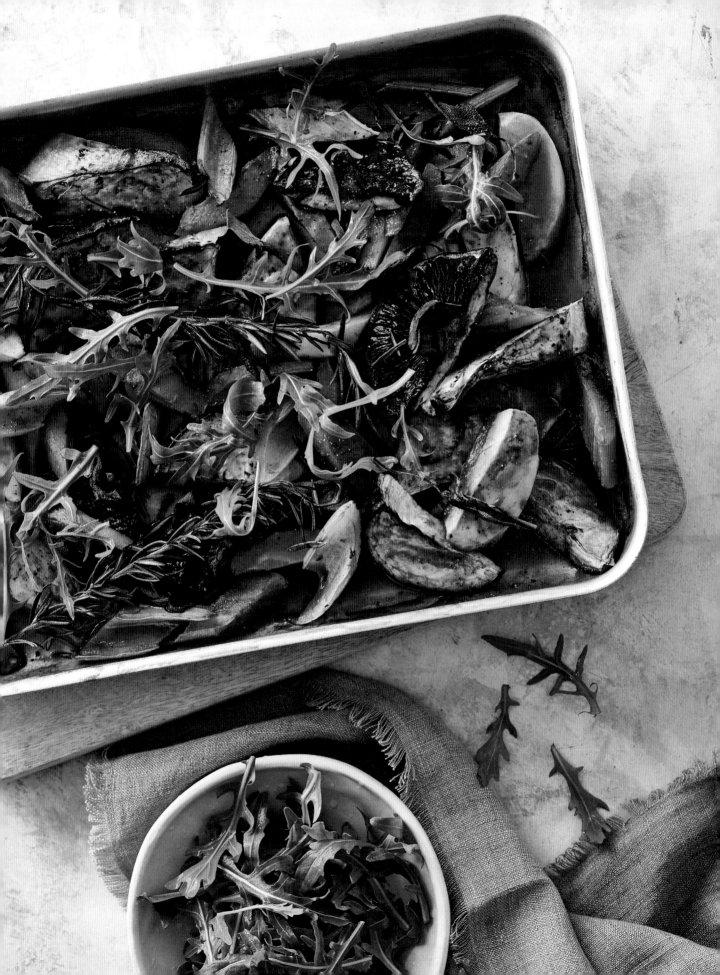

Hearty roast vegetables

Preparation: 15 minutes, plus standing time ✳ **Cooking:** 35 minutes
Difficulty: Easy

2 tablespoons salt-reduced tomato paste
1 cup (250 ml) salt-reduced
    vegetable stock
1 eggplant, coarsely chopped
500 g mixed mushrooms (such as
    Swiss brown, portobello and button),
    wiped clean, halved if large
2 small swedes, peeled
    and coarsely chopped
2 carrots, halved lengthways
    and thickly sliced diagonally
4 sticks celery, thickly sliced diagonally
1 bunch sage, leaves picked
2 sprigs rosemary
100 g rocket leaves

Preheat the oven to 220°C (200°C fan-forced).

Combine the tomato paste and stock in the base of a heavy-based baking dish. Add the eggplant, mushroom, swede, carrot, celery, sage and rosemary, season with freshly ground black pepper, then toss in the stock mixture to coat.

Bake for 35 minutes or until the vegetables are cooked and the sauce has thickened. Remove the dish from the oven and stand for 10 minutes, then add the rocket and toss well to combine. Serve hot, warm or at room temperature.

UNITS PER SERVE Grains **0** ✳ Meat and alternatives **0** ✳ Fruit **0** ✳ Vegetables **4** ✳ Dairy **0** ✳ Fats and oils **0**

Creamy cauliflower and swede soup

Preparation: 15 minutes ✳ **Cooking:** 20 minutes
Difficulty: Easy

SERVES 4

3 cups (300 g) cauliflower florets

2 swedes, peeled and finely chopped

2 zucchini, chopped

1 large leek, white part only, trimmed, halved lengthways and thinly sliced

1 litre salt-reduced vegetable stock

2 tablespoons thyme leaves

Combine the cauliflower, swede, zucchini, leek and stock in a large saucepan over medium heat. Cook, partially covered and stirring occasionally, for 20 minutes or until the vegetables are very soft.

Using a hand-held blender, blend the soup in the pan until completely smooth. Season with freshly ground black pepper. Divide the soup among serving bowls, sprinkle with thyme leaves and serve.

UNITS PER SERVE Grains **0** ✳ Meat and alternatives **0** ✳ Fruit **0** ✳ Vegetables **3.5** ✳ Dairy **0** ✳ Fats and oils **0**

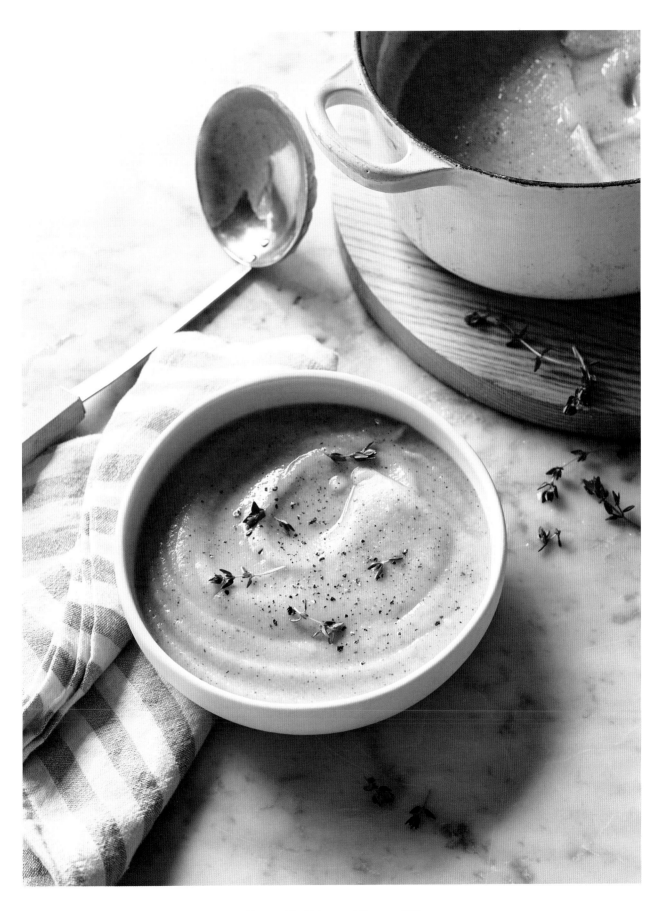

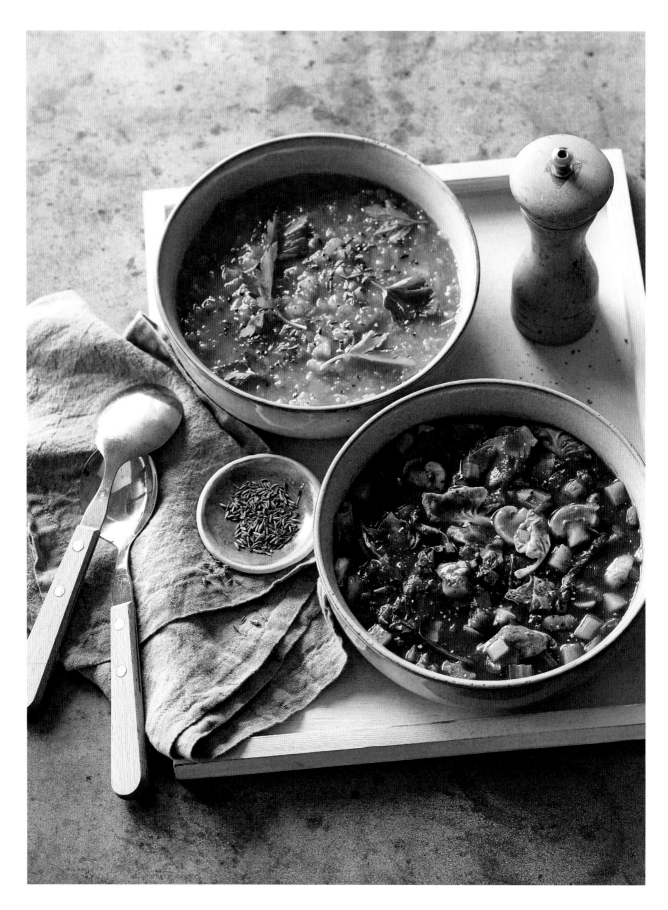

Winter vegetable soup

Preparation: 15 minutes
Cooking: 25 minutes
Difficulty: Easy

SERVES 4

2 tablespoons salt-reduced tomato paste

2 teaspoons dried Italian herbs

3 cloves garlic, crushed

1 x 400 g tin crushed tomatoes

1 litre salt-reduced vegetable stock

1 red onion, chopped

1 swede (about 300 g), peeled and finely chopped

2 sticks celery, chopped

250 g button mushrooms, thickly sliced

200 g Brussels sprouts, trimmed

1 bunch English spinach, leaves picked

Combine the tomato paste, herbs, garlic and tomatoes in a large saucepan over high heat. Cook, stirring, for 5 minutes or until reduced and thickened.

Reduce the heat to medium. Add the stock, onion, swede, celery, mushroom and sprouts. Cook, stirring occasionally, for 20 minutes or until the vegetables are tender. Add the spinach and stir until wilted. Season with freshly ground black pepper and serve.

Mashed pumpkin soup

Preparation: 15 minutes
Cooking: 25 minutes
Difficulty: Easy

SERVES 4

500 g peeled, seeded butternut pumpkin, chopped

2 carrots, chopped

2 sticks celery, finely chopped

1 large onion, finely chopped

1 litre salt-reduced vegetable stock

1 tablespoon cumin seeds

2 tablespoons chopped flat-leaf parsley

Combine the pumpkin, carrot, celery, onion and stock in a large saucepan over medium heat. Cook, partially covered and stirring occasionally, for 20 minutes or until the vegetables are very soft.

Remove the pan from the heat. Using a vegetable masher, mash together until well combined and the vegetables are nicely broken up. Season with freshly ground black pepper, then cover and set aside to keep warm.

Place a small non-stick frying pan over medium heat. Add the cumin seeds and toast, shaking the pan occasionally, for 1–2 minutes or until fragrant and lightly golden.

Divide the pumpkin soup among serving bowls, sprinkle with the toasted cumin seeds and parsley, and serve.

UNITS PER SERVE Grains **0** ✳ Meat and alternatives **0**
Fruit **0** ✳ Vegetables **5** ✳ Dairy **0** ✳ Fats and oils **0**

UNITS PER SERVE Grains **0** ✳ Meat and alternatives **0**
Fruit **0** ✳ Vegetables **3** ✳ Dairy **0** ✳ Fats and oils **0**

Simple spring soup

Preparation: 15 minutes ☀ **Cooking:** 15 minutes
Difficulty: Easy

SERVES 4

2 cloves garlic, thinly sliced

2 bulbs baby fennel, trimmed, cored
and finely chopped

2 zucchini, peeled into long thin ribbons

1 bunch broccolini, trimmed
and thinly sliced

1 litre salt-reduced vegetable stock

1 cup (120 g) frozen peas

1 bunch asparagus, trimmed
and thinly sliced

2 spring onions, white and green parts
thinly sliced

1 cup basil leaves

Combine the garlic, fennel, zucchini, broccolini and stock in a large saucepan over medium heat. Cook, stirring occasionally, for 10 minutes.

Add the peas, asparagus and spring onion and cook, stirring, for 2 minutes. Season with freshly ground black pepper.

Divide the soup among bowls, top with basil leaves and serve.

UNITS PER SERVE Grains **0** ☀ Meat and alternatives **0** ☀ Fruit **0** ☀ Vegetables **4** ☀ Dairy **0** ☀ Fats and oils **0**

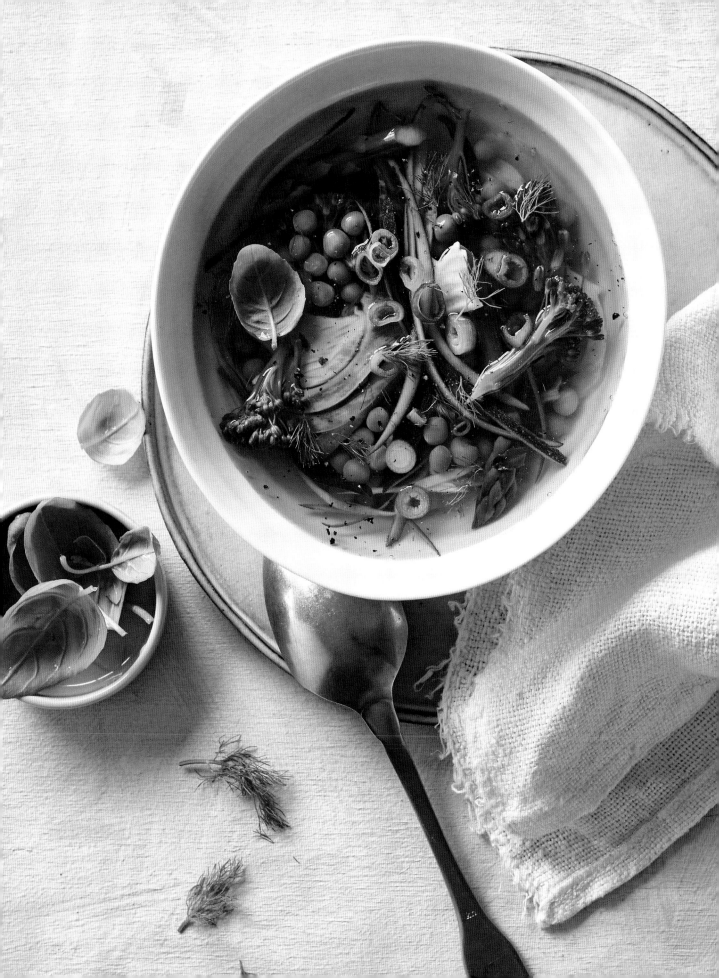

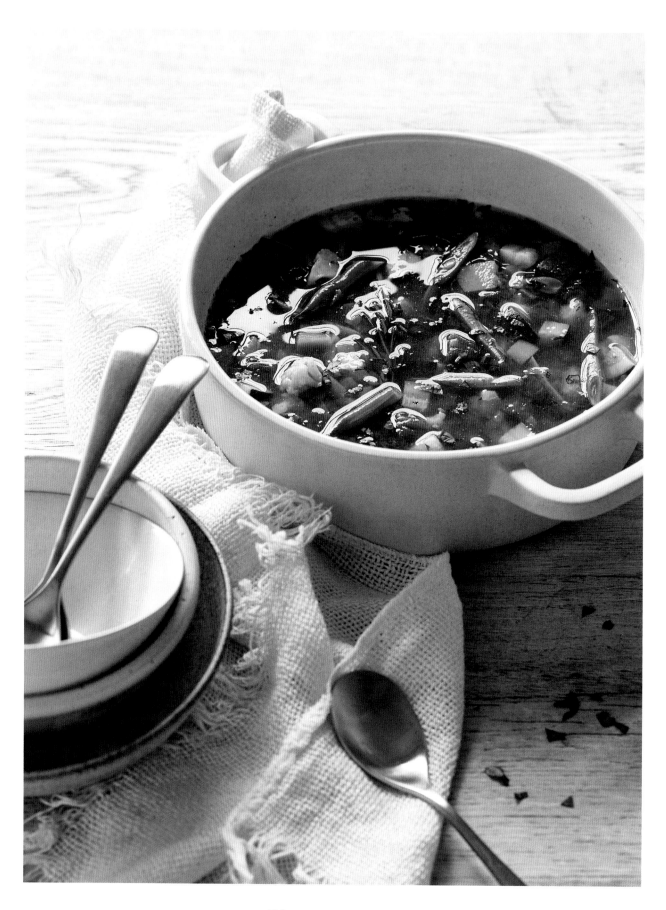

End-of-the-week soup

Preparation: 15 minutes ✳ **Cooking:** 20 minutes
Difficulty: Easy

1 clove garlic, finely chopped
2 cm piece ginger, finely chopped
1 onion, chopped
100 g peeled, seeded butternut
   pumpkin, chopped
1 zucchini, chopped
2 over-ripe tomatoes, chopped
½ cup (50 g) chopped cauliflower
   florets and stems
50 g green beans, trimmed and chopped
½ bunch flat-leaf parsley,
   leaves and stems finely chopped
1 sprig rosemary
1 litre salt-reduced vegetable stock

Place all the ingredients in a large saucepan over medium heat. Cook, stirring occasionally, for 20 minutes or until the vegetables are very tender.

Season with freshly ground black pepper and serve.

NOTE

Feel free to use any leftover vegetables you have in your fridge for this versatile soup. Soft veg, such as snow peas or spinach, should be added in the last 5 minutes of cooking time so they don't overcook.

UNITS PER SERVE Grains **0** ✳ Meat and alternatives **0** ✳ Fruit **0** ✳ Vegetables **3** ✳ Dairy **0** ✳ Fats and oils **0**

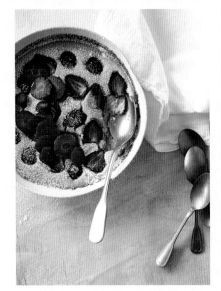

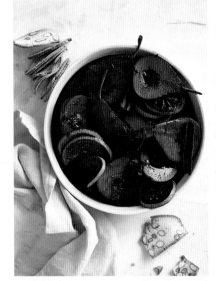

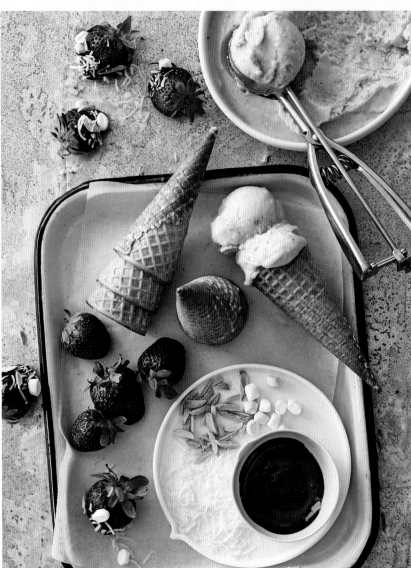

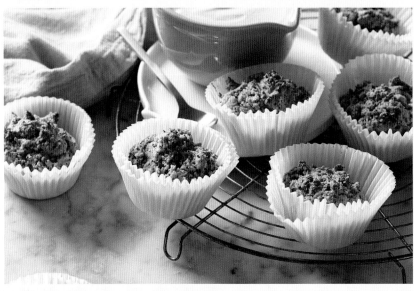

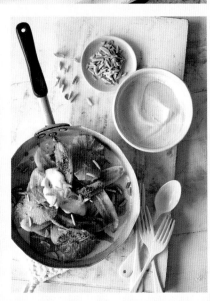

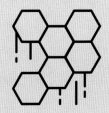

7. Healthy Indulgences

Caramelised orange bananas with brandy yoghurt

Preparation: 20 minutes ✳ **Cooking:** 10 minutes
Difficulty: Easy

SERVES 4

2 navel oranges
500 g low-fat natural Greek-style yoghurt
1 tablespoon brown sugar
¼ cup (60 ml) brandy
2 tablespoons light margarine
2 teaspoons vanilla
4 bananas, peeled and halved lengthways
28 g flaked almonds, toasted

Finely grate the zest of one of the oranges and place in a bowl. Remove and discard the peel and white pith from both oranges, then slice into 3 mm thick rounds. Set aside.

Add the yoghurt, sugar and 1 tablespoon brandy to the orange zest in the bowl and mix well to combine. Cover and chill until ready to serve.

Melt half the margarine in a large non-stick heavy-based frying pan over high heat. Add half the vanilla, half the orange slices and half the banana slices. Cook, turning occasionally, for 2–3 minutes or until golden. Transfer to a plate. Repeat with the remaining margarine, vanilla, orange and banana. Remove the pan from the heat and add the remaining brandy, stirring well until bubbling and all the flavours are released from the base of the pan.

Divide the brandy yoghurt among four bowls. Top with the warm orange and banana and pour over the brandy mixture from the pan. Sprinkle with the toasted almonds and serve warm.

UNITS PER SERVE Fruit **1** ✳ Indulgence **2**

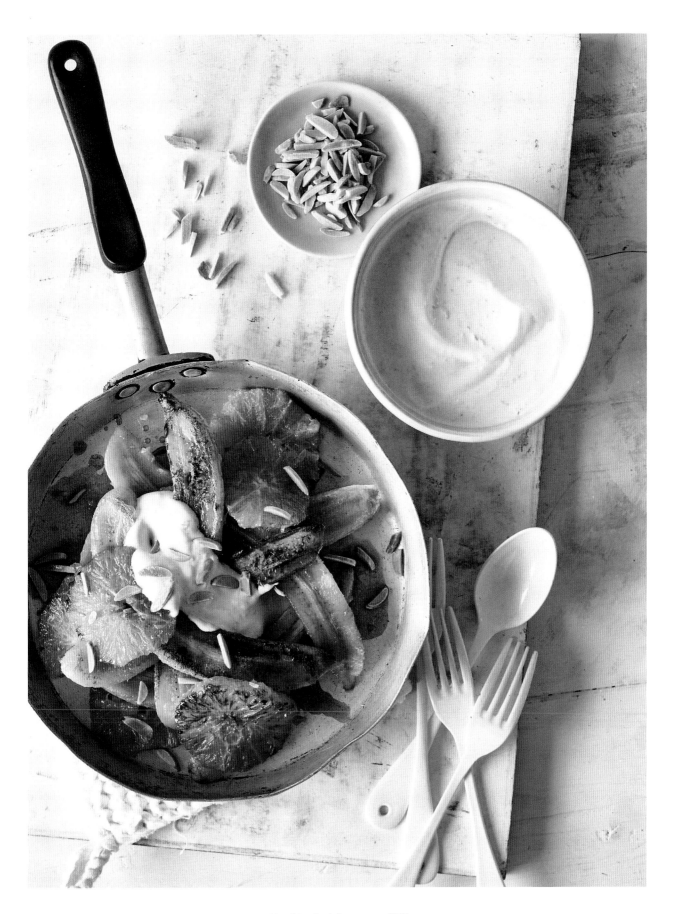

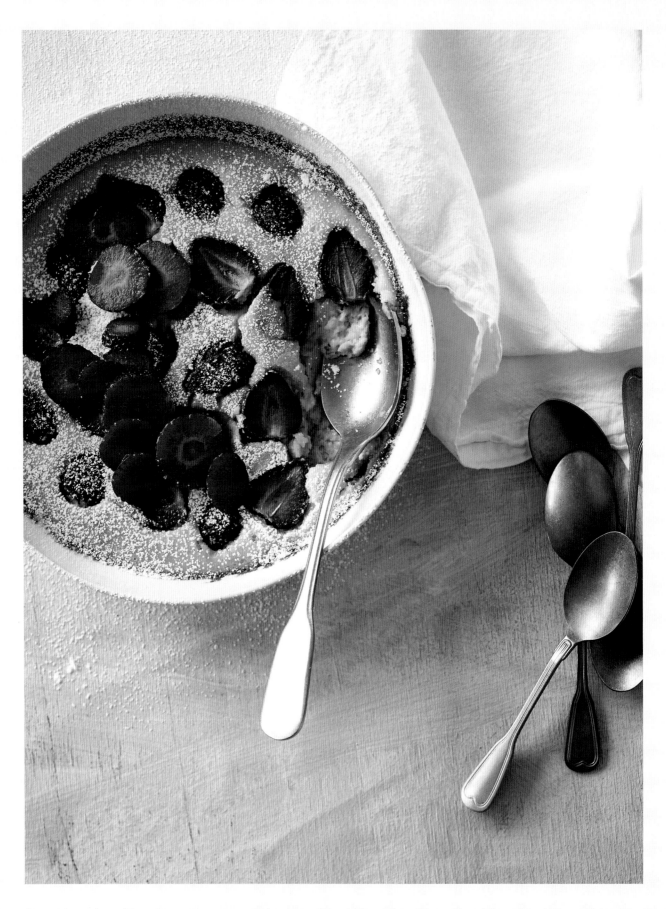

Strawberry clafoutis

Preparation: 20 minutes * **Cooking:** 25 minutes
Difficulty: Easy

SERVES 4

light olive oil spray, for cooking
250 g strawberries, hulled and halved
⅓ cup (40 g) almond meal
2 tablespoons caster sugar
¾ cup (180 ml) low-fat milk
2 large eggs
1 teaspoon vanilla
icing sugar, for dusting
1 cup low-fat vanilla custard, to serve

Preheat the oven to 180°C (160°C fan-forced). Lightly spray a 20 cm shallow glass pie plate with olive oil. Scatter 200 g of the strawberries evenly over the base.

Combine the almond meal and caster sugar in a bowl. Whisk together the milk, eggs and vanilla in a large jug, then slowly add to the almond mixture, whisking constantly until smooth and well combined.

Carefully pour the batter over the strawberries in the pie plate. Bake for 25 minutes or until just set in the centre. Leave to stand for 5 minutes, then dust with icing sugar and scatter over the reserved strawberries. Serve immediately with vanilla custard.

UNITS PER SERVE Fruit **0** * Indulgence **2**

Mango banana nice-cream cones

Preparation: 20 minutes,
plus freezing time
Cooking: nil
Difficulty: Easy

SERVES 4

2 mangoes, peeled and chopped
4 ripe bananas, peeled and chopped
250 g low-fat berry yoghurt
4 waffle cones

Line a large baking tray with baking paper. Arrange the fruit on the tray in a single layer and freeze for 3–4 hours or until firm.

Transfer the frozen fruit to an upright blender and add the yoghurt. Blend on high speed, scraping down the sides of the jug occasionally, until completely smooth. Serve immediately scooped into cones.

NOTES

If the mixture is too thick and won't blend easily, just add 1–2 tablespoons water to help loosen it.

UNITS PER SERVE Fruit **1.5** ✳ Indulgence **1**

Rocky road strawberries

Preparation: 15 minutes,
plus chilling time
Cooking: 5 minutes
Difficulty: Easy

SERVES 8

100 g dark chocolate (70% cocoa solids), chopped
1 tablespoon shredded coconut
8 mini pink and white marshmallows, quartered
1 tablespoon slivered almonds, toasted
8 extra-large strawberries

Place the chocolate in a small heatproof bowl set over a small saucepan of gently simmering water, making sure the base of the bowl does not touch the water. Stir for 1–2 minutes or until the chocolate is melted and smooth. Remove from the heat, keeping the bowl over the saucepan.

Line a large baking tray with baking paper.

Combine the coconut, marshmallow and almonds in a small bowl.

Using their green tops to hold, dip one strawberry at a time into the melted chocolate, then immediately dip into the coconut mixture to coat. Place on the prepared tray. Chill for 20 minutes or until set firm. Serve chilled.

UNITS PER SERVE Fruit **0** ✳ Indulgence **1**

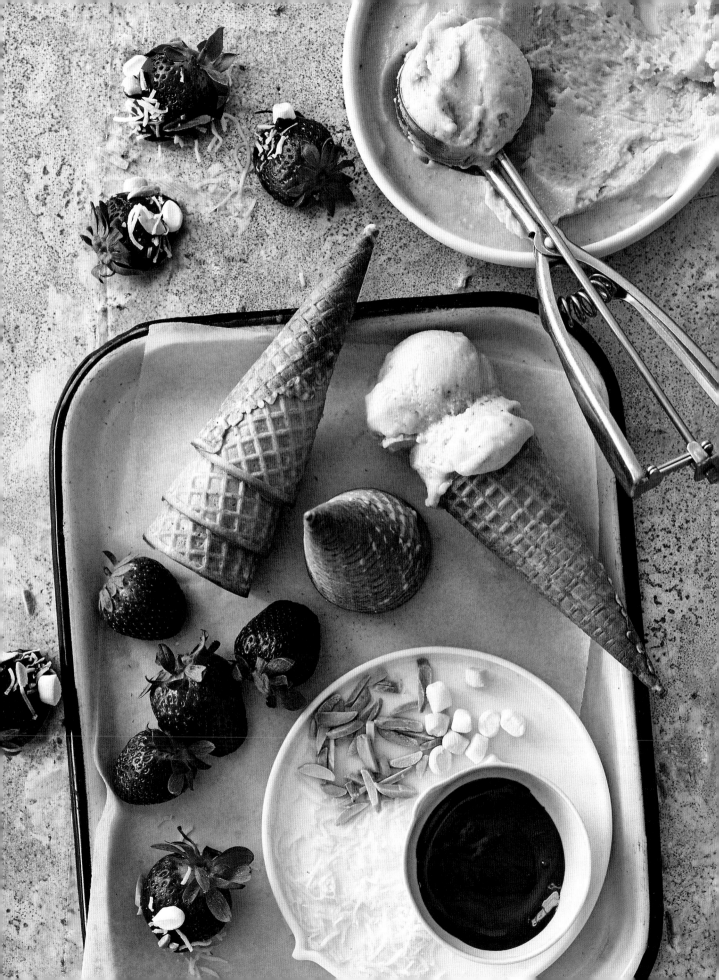

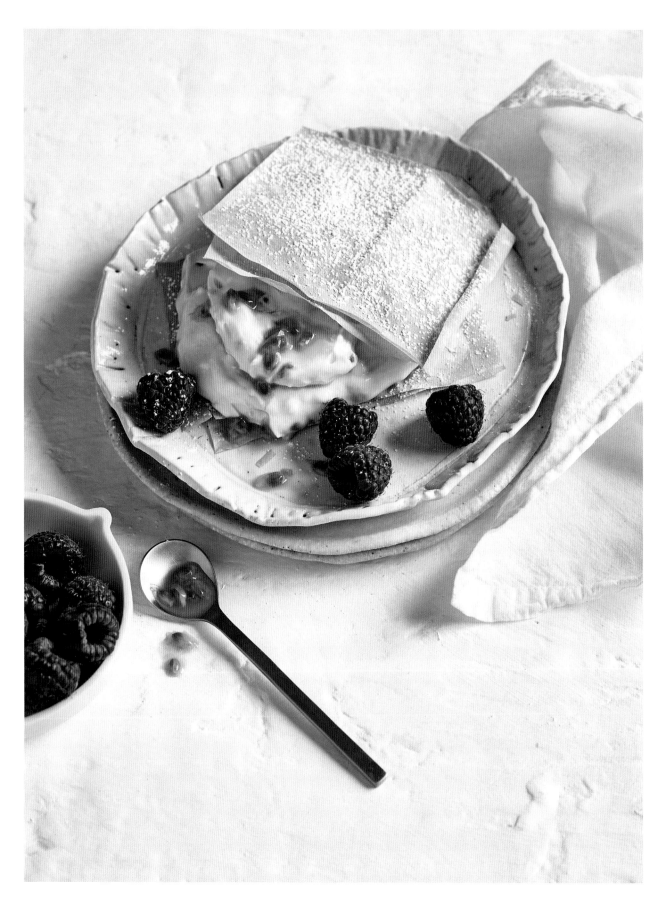

Passionfruit custard and raspberry stacks

Preparation: 30 minutes, plus cooling time ✳ **Cooking:** 20 minutes
Difficulty: Easy

SERVES 4

2 sheets filo pastry
light olive oil spray, for cooking
1 teaspoon icing sugar
1 cup (250 ml) low-fat vanilla custard
250 g light cream cheese,
    at room temperature
4 passionfruit, halved, seeds and
    juice scraped (you'll need ⅓ cup
    seeds and juice)
250 g raspberries

Preheat the oven to 180°C (160°C fan-forced) and line two large baking trays with baking paper.

Place one sheet of filo on a clean work surface and lightly spray with olive oil. Place the other sheet of filo directly on top of the first and lightly spray with olive oil. Cut the stack lengthways into thirds, then cut each third crossways into four pieces to make 12 pieces. Transfer to the prepared trays.

Bake the filo for 20 minutes or until cooked and golden, swapping the trays halfway through. Remove and cool on the trays. Lightly dust the tops with the icing sugar.

Place the custard and cream cheese in a bowl. Using a hand-held electric mixer, beat on high speed until completely smooth. Beat in three-quarters of the passionfruit seeds and juice until well combined, reserving the rest to garnish.

Set out four plates and place a piece of filo, icing sugar-side up, on each. Spoon over half the custard mixture and dot with some of the raspberries. Place another piece of filo on top, then spoon over the remaining custard mixture and dot with some more raspberries. Finish the stacks with the remaining filo pieces, spoon over the reserved passionfruit seeds and juice and scatter with the remaining raspberries. Serve immediately.

NOTES

This is a great sweet treat to prep the day before serving. Store the cooled filo pieces in an airtight container at room temperature and the custard mixture in an airtight container in the fridge. Take the custard out of the fridge about 20 minutes before using so it softens slightly.

UNITS PER SERVE Fruit **0.5** ✳ Indulgence **2**

Dark choc and date loaf

Preparation: 20 minutes, plus resting time ✳ **Cooking:** 1 hour
Difficulty: Easy

SERVES 10

2 over-ripe bananas, peeled and chopped

2 tablespoons pure maple syrup

½ cup (100 g) unsweetened apple puree

1 large egg, lightly whisked

1 teaspoon ground cinnamon

2 cups (320 g) wholemeal
self-raising flour

50 g dark chocolate (70% cocoa solids),
chopped

8 large fresh dates, pitted and chopped

Preheat the oven to 180°C (160°C fan-forced). Line the base and sides of an 18 cm x 10 cm loaf tin with baking paper.

Place the banana in a large bowl and mash until smooth. Add the remaining ingredients and stir until well combined. Spoon the mixture into the prepared tin and level the surface.

Bake for 1 hour or until golden and a skewer inserted in the centre comes out clean. Cool in the tin for 10 minutes, then turn out and cut into 10 even slices. Serve warm.

NOTES

The cooled loaf can be stored in an airtight container in the fridge for up to 1 week; toast to warm and crisp up before serving. Slices of the cooled loaf can be wrapped individually and frozen for up to 3 months; thaw in the fridge overnight and toast to warm and crisp up before serving.

UNITS PER SERVE Fruit **0** ✳ Indulgence **1.5**

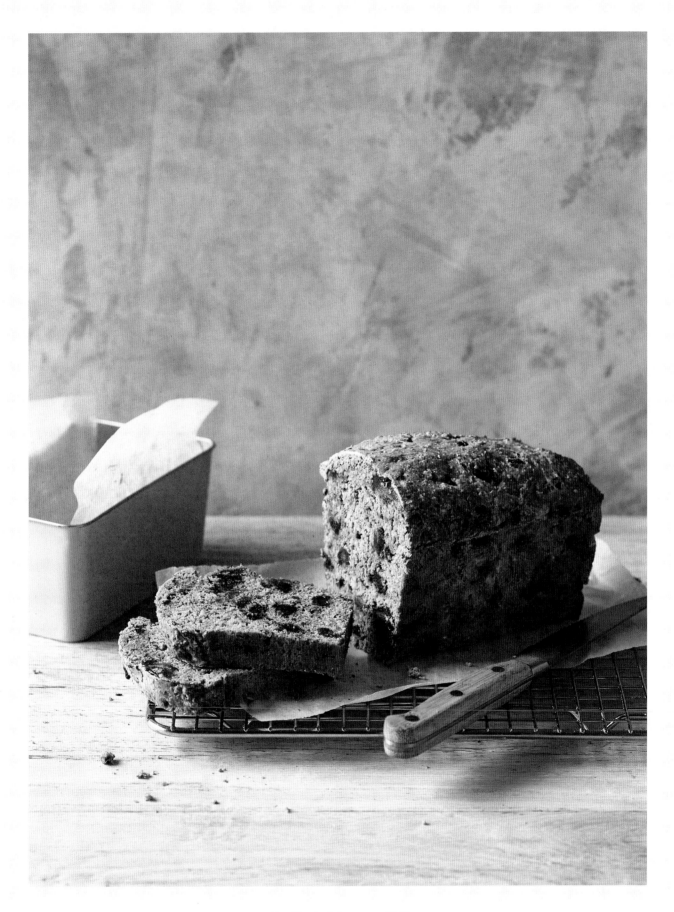

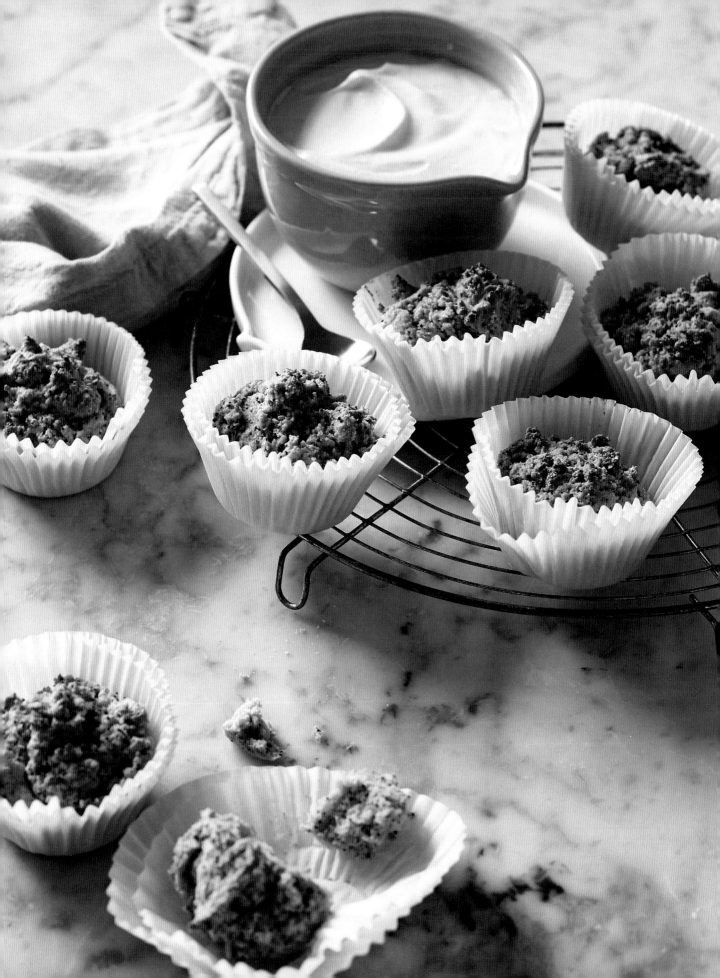

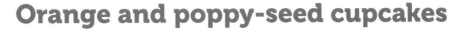

Orange and poppy-seed cupcakes

Preparation: 20 minutes ✳ **Cooking:** 15 minutes
Difficulty: Easy

SERVES 12

1 orange, peel and white pith removed,
    flesh chopped
1 tablespoon honey
2 teaspoons vanilla
½ cup (100 g) unsweetened apple puree
2 large eggs, lightly whisked
2 cups (320 g) wholemeal
    self-raising flour
1 tablespoon poppy seeds
low-fat vanilla yoghurt, to serve
    (optional)

Preheat the oven to 180°C (160°C fan-forced). Line a 12-hole, ⅓ cup muffin tin with paper patty cases.

Place the orange, honey, vanilla and apple puree in an upright blender and blend on high speed until completely smooth. Transfer to a bowl.

Add the egg, flour and poppy seeds to the orange mixture and stir gently until just combined – do not overmix or the cupcakes will be tough. Divide the batter evenly among the prepared muffin holes.

Bake for 15 minutes or until golden and a skewer inserted in the centre of a cupcake comes out clean. Cool in the tin for 3 minutes, then remove and serve warm with a small dollop of yoghurt, if desired.

NOTES

The cooled cupcakes can be stored in an airtight container at room temperature for up to 2 days, in the fridge for up to 5 days, or wrapped individually and frozen for up to 3 months (just thaw them in the fridge overnight). Chilled cupcakes can be gently reheated in the microwave on medium–high for 5–10 seconds.

UNITS PER SERVE Fruit **0** ✳ Indulgence **2**

Upside-down blueberry cheesecakes

Preparation: 15 minutes ✻ **Cooking:** nil
Difficulty: Easy

SERVES 6

250 g spreadable light cream cheese

500 g fresh reduced-fat ricotta

1 tablespoon honey

2 teaspoons vanilla

300 g low-fat strawberry dairy dessert
(e.g. Fruche fromage frais)

250 g blueberries

2 savoiardi biscuits, crumbled

Place the cream cheese, ricotta, honey and vanilla in a large bowl. Using an electric hand-held mixer, beat on high speed until smooth and well combined. Fold in the dairy dessert and half the blueberries.

Divide half the remaining blueberries among four 250 ml glass tumblers. Top evenly with the cream-cheese mixture and sprinkle over the biscuit crumbs. Scatter over the remaining blueberries and serve immediately.

NOTES

These cheesecakes can be made up to 1 day ahead of time; just cover and keep chilled until you are ready to serve, adding the biscuit crumbs just before serving.

UNITS PER SERVE Fruit **0.5** ✻ Indulgence **2**

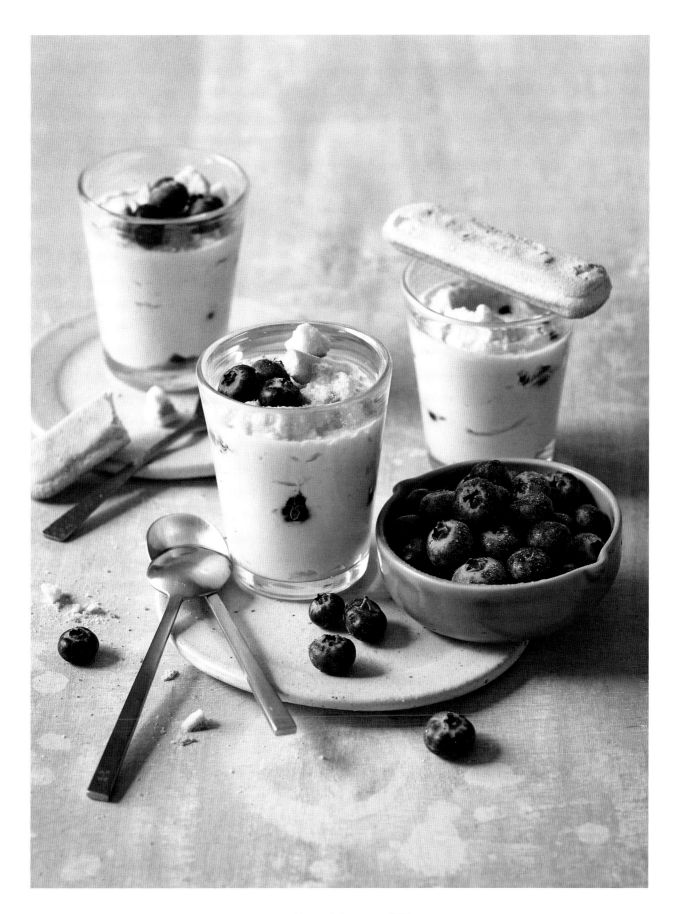

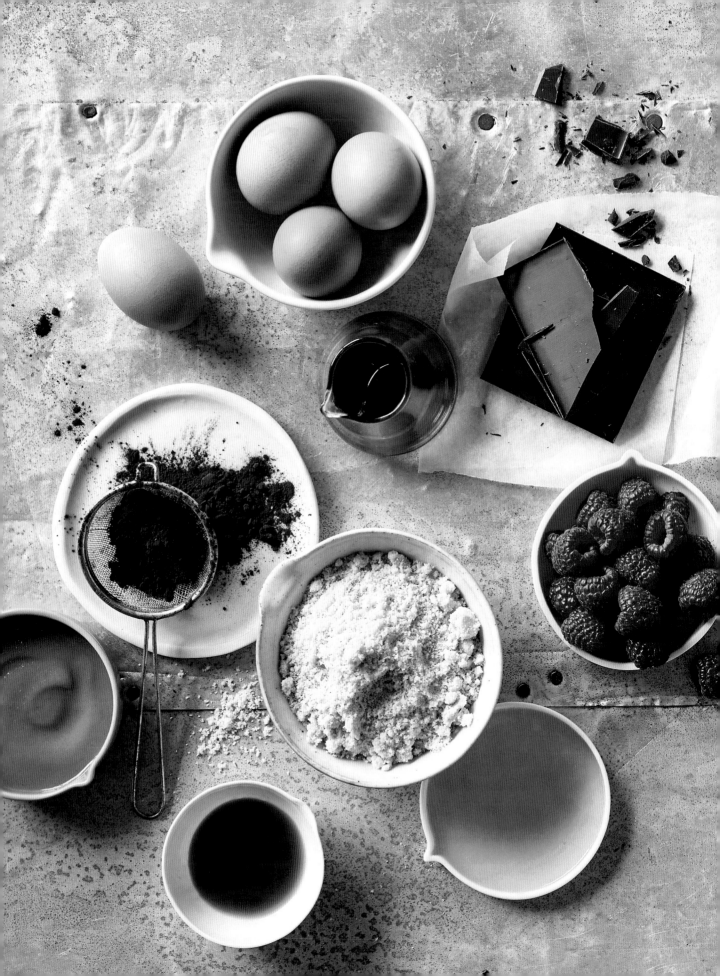

Double-choc raspberry brownie

Preparation: 20 minutes, plus cooling time ✻ **Cooking:** 35 minutes
Difficulty: Easy

SERVES 8

¼ cup (45 g) light margarine, melted

½ cup (50 g) cocoa powder

¼ cup (50 g) unsweetened apple puree

2 tablespoons pure maple syrup

2 teaspoons vanilla

4 large eggs

1 cup (120 g) almond meal

100 g dark chocolate (70% cocoa solids), broken into pieces

125 g raspberries

Preheat the oven to 160°C (140°C fan-forced). Line the base and sides of a 20 cm square cake tin with baking paper.

Place the melted margarine, cocoa powder, apple puree, maple syrup, vanilla and eggs in a large bowl. Using a hand-held electric mixer, beat on high speed until smooth and well combined. Stir in the almond meal.

Pour the almond mixture into the prepared tin and smooth the surface. Gently press the chocolate and raspberries into the batter until partially submerged. Bake for 30–35 minutes or until the brownie is set around the edges and just set in the centre. Cool completely in the tin. Cut into 8 even pieces and serve.

NOTES

You can swap the fresh raspberries for ¾ cup (95 g) frozen raspberries, if desired.

The cooled brownies can be stored in an airtight container at room temperature for up to 3 days, in the fridge for up to 1 week, or in the freezer up to 3 months. Thaw overnight in the fridge.

UNITS PER SERVE

Fruit **0** ✻ Indulgence **2**

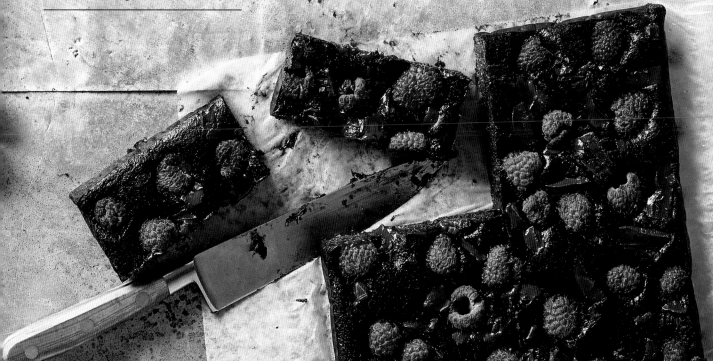

Mulled wine pears

Preparation: 20 minutes ✻ **Cooking:** 25 minutes
Difficulty: Easy

SERVES 4

3 cups (750 ml) red wine of choice

2 cinnamon sticks, broken in half

4 cloves

2 star anise

1 orange, sliced into 5 mm thick rounds

1 small lemon, sliced into 5 mm
    thick rounds

4 firm green pears, peeled,
    halved lengthways and cored

8 thin pistachio biscotti, to serve

VANILLA RICOTTA

1 cup (200 g) fresh ricotta

125 g low-fat vanilla yoghurt

2 teaspoons vanilla

Combine the wine, cinnamon sticks, cloves, star anise, orange and lemon slices in a large deep heavy-based frying pan over low–medium heat. Add the pears and bring to a gentle simmer, then reduce the heat to low and cook, carefully turning the pears occasionally, for 20 minutes or until the pears are just tender and the mulled wine has reduced slightly.

Meanwhile, to make the vanilla ricotta, use a hand-held electric mixer to beat all the ingredients until very smooth and well combined. Cover and store in the fridge until ready to serve.

Spoon the pears and mulled wine into serving bowls. Serve warm with vanilla ricotta and biscotti.

UNITS PER SERVE Fruit **1.5** ✻ Indulgence **1**

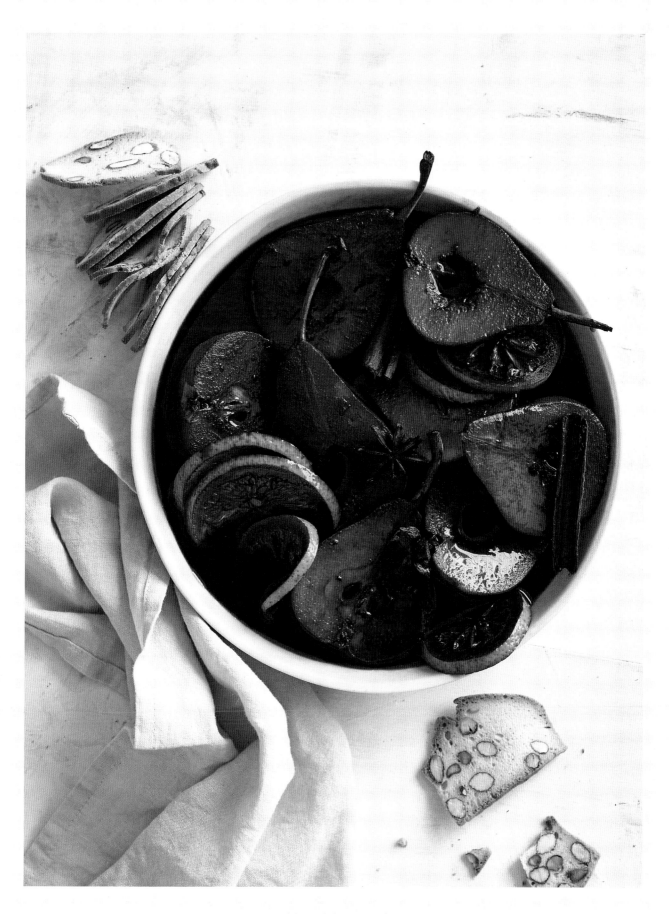

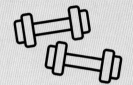

PART FOUR

Resistance Exercises

Our resistance exercise program

Whether you wish to lose weight, control your weight, reduce your body fat or increase your muscle mass and strength, this program is a practical and easy-to-implement home-based training routine that will help you achieve these goals.

Before starting any new exercise program, particularly if you have not undertaken much physical activity in recent times, it is a good idea to talk with your doctor, allied health or exercise professional to discuss any medical conditions or physical issues you need to consider, and to ensure it is safe for you to commence exercise. An accredited exercise physiologist or fitness professional can also help you to tailor an exercise program to meet your individual needs and abilities.

What is resistance training?

Resistance training is based on the principle that the muscles of your body will work to overcome a force of resistance when they are required to do so. When you undertake resistance training repeatedly and consistently, you get stronger and your muscles can become bigger.

Our resistance exercise training program is based on the principles and formats that research studies have shown will effectively improve body composition (by reducing body fat and increasing muscle mass), and increase muscle strength, when combined with the protein intake plan set out in this book.

Types of resistance training

There are many types of resistance exercise training that can be performed to overload the muscles of the body. These include using your own body weight, free weights such as dumbbells or barbells, weight machines, medicine (weighted) balls and resistance bands.

This program has been designed with a mix of exercises that use body weight and dumbbells, to make them convenient to do at home with minimal expense.

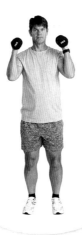

Using the exercise program

Before you get started, here are the basic principles and concepts to help you get the most from your resistance exercise training.

* **Frequency**: We recommend performing two–three resistance exercise training sessions per week on non-consecutive days. As a good rule of thumb, rest a muscle group for up to 48 hours before working the same muscle group again, to allow time for the muscle to repair and adapt after a workout.
* **Duration**: Each exercise session should last 45–60 minutes.
* **Exercises and body region target**: Aim for a whole-body workout. Research shows improvements in body composition and strength are greater in people who train all body parts (arms, legs and trunk) than those who only perform specific body-region exercises. To achieve a whole-body workout in each session, perform eight–ten exercises in each workout that will train the major muscle groups across the whole body, by including three–four upper body exercises, three–four lower body exercises, and at least two core body exercises from the options presented.
* **Repetitions**: This is the number of times you continuously repeat each exercise in a set. To maximise gains in muscle strength and size, aim to perform 8–15 repetitions of an exercise in each set.
* **Set**: A set refers to a group of repetitions performed without resting. For example, two sets of push-ups with 15 reps means that you do 15 push-ups, then rest your muscles and do another 15 push-ups. At each exercise session, aim to perform two–four sets of each exercise. Remember that for exercises such as the side lunge (page 256), where you exercise each side of the body separately, you will need to perform the exercise on both sides of your body to count as one completed set. If you are just beginning, start with one set of each exercise, and gradually build up to more sets on subsequent sessions.
* **Intensity and progressive overload**: To get the most from your exercise program, the resistance load (i.e. weight) needs to be heavy enough to sufficiently overload the muscle, but not so heavy that you lose your technique and increase your risk of injury. As already mentioned, to maximise gains in muscle strength and size, it is recommended you perform 8–15 repetitions for each set. A number of experts have shown that if you work to the point where your effort is 8–9/10 by your last repetition, you're going to get the benefits we've outlined (see the rating of perceived exertion scale on page 246). As you progress and become stronger, increase the number of repetitions you perform in each set. Once you can comfortably do 12–15 reps, you need to increase the load (weight) so that you can only do eight repetitions to fatigue again. This will ensure your muscles continue to adapt and get stronger, so that you fully benefit from the exercise program.
* **Pace and tempo**: Perform each exercise at a good pace, using a 2:1:2 tempo (effort:hold:release). For example, for the dumbbell (bicep) curl (see page 248), this would mean taking 2 seconds to lift the dumbbell to your shoulder; holding the dumbbell at the top for 1 second; then taking 2 seconds to return the dumbbell to the starting position.
* **Breathing**: It is important to remember to not hold your breath while doing the exercises. Aim to breathe out during the effort phase (when the muscle is shortening under tension, such as when you are lifting a dumbbell), and breathe in during the release phase (when the muscle is lengthening under tension, such as when you are lowering a dumbbell).
* **Rest**: As this program is designed to fatigue the muscles you are working, you need to rest between sets. Allow 1–2 minutes between sets for recovery.
* **Variation**: To maintain improvement, variety and to keep it interesting, vary your training program every 6–8 weeks. You can do this by increasing the number of sets, repetitions and intensity (size of the weight used), varying the exercises undertaken or changing the frequency of sessions and rests between sets. If you keep doing the same thing for an extended period, your muscles will get used to the workout and will stop adapting. So, change your workout every 6–8 weeks to keep your muscles guessing!

Research suggests that expert supervision and instruction from a certified fitness professional can improve your results as it will enable you to safely perform more complex exercises using the proper technique. If you experience any pain or discomfort during your exercise sessions, contact a health professional before progressing with your program.

Aerobic exercise training

In addition to resistance training, aerobic exercise (also known as endurance exercise or cardiorespiratory fitness training) is recommended to improve health and wellbeing.

Aerobic exercise involves sustained activities that use large muscle groups in a rhythmic manner, such as walking, running, rowing, cycling and swimming. While the effects of aerobic exercise training on muscle mass and strength is less certain compared to the clear effects of resistance exercise training, it does deliver numerous health benefits. These include improvements in:

* insulin sensitivity
* blood glucose control
* blood cholesterol levels
* physical function
* aerobic fitness, which reduces the risk of premature death from all causes.

Aerobic exercise training also:

* reduces blood pressure
* increases energy expenditure, to assist in weight control
* reduces the risk of some cancers, including colon and breast cancer.

Any comprehensive physical activity and lifestyle program should include some aerobic exercise training. Aim for at least three aerobic exercise sessions per week, of moderate or higher (vigorous) intensity. The chart below can help you keep track of the relative intensity of your workout. A moderate intensity corresponds to a rating of 3 on this scale.

Ideally, try to complete these aerobic exercise sessions on alternate days to your resistance exercises, which is also a good way to mix up your routine to keep it interesting. Your aerobic sessions could include activities such as brisk walking, jogging, cycling, rowing, aerobics and swimming, for a duration of 45–60 minutes each session. However, if you are only starting out, it is best to begin with shorter sessions of about 30 minutes and build up progressively over several weeks.

Rating of perceived exertion of exercise session

0	Rest
1	Very, very easy
2	Easy
3	Moderate
4	Somewhat hard
5	Hard
6	–
7	Very hard
8	–
9	–
10	Maximum

Your resistance training program

You can build your own exercise program by selecting 8–10 exercises from the following pages, choosing a minimum of three exercises from the upper body options, three exercises from the lower body options, and at least two exercises from the core or trunk options.

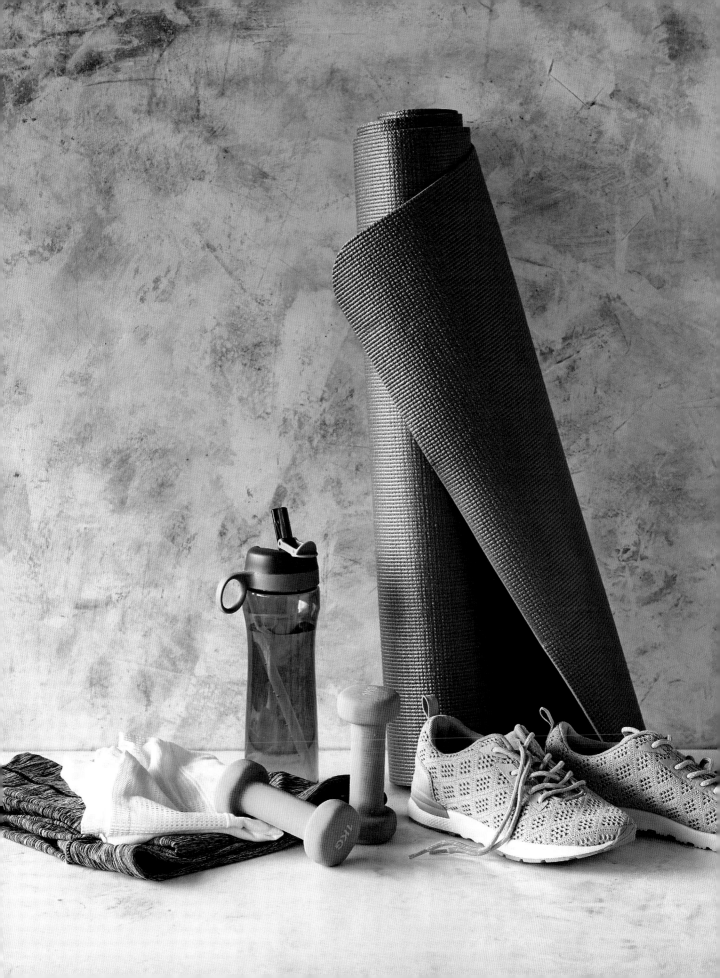

UPPER BODY

Standing dumbbell (bicep) curl

Muscles: Front upper arm (biceps) ✳ **Weight:** Dumbbells

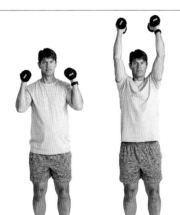

Start Stand tall with your feet shoulder-width apart and your arms by your sides, with a dumbbell in each hand hanging by your thighs, palms facing forward.

Action » Keeping your elbows tucked and your upper arms locked in place, curl the dumbbells as close to your shoulders as you can. Avoid swinging your body to lift the dumbbells. If you find you need to do this, decrease the weights until you become stronger.

» Pause, then slowly lower the weights back to the starting position.

Shoulder press

Muscles: Shoulders (deltoid) ✳ **Weight:** Dumbbells

Start Stand tall with your feet hip-width apart, and hold a pair of dumbbells just above your shoulders, with your elbows tucked and palms facing each other.

Action » Press the weights directly above your shoulders until your arms are straight and your biceps are next to your ears.

» Pause, then lower the weights back to the starting position.

Lateral shoulder fly

Muscles: Shoulders (deltoid) ✳ **Weight:** Dumbbells

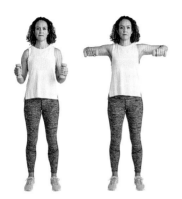

Start Stand tall with your feet shoulder-width apart and your arms by your sides, with a dumbbell in each hand. Hold your elbows close to your torso, with your palms facing your thighs. Bend your elbows at a 90-degree angle, with your palms facing each other inwards.

Action » Keeping your torso still, lift your upper arms outwards and upwards while maintaining the 90-degree elbow bend, until your arms are parallel to the floor and your palms are facing downwards.

» Pause, then lower the dumbbells back to the starting position.

Push-up

Muscles: Chest/upper arm (pectoral/triceps) ✳ **Weight:** Body

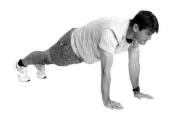

Start   With your hands shoulder-width apart (fingers pointing forward), and keeping your feet flexed at hip-distance apart, tighten your core, with your knees, hips and shoulders in a straight line (this is the plank position).

Action   » Lower your upper body by bending the elbows outwards, until your chest reaches an inch or two above the floor.

       » Pause, then push back up until your arms are straight, keeping your elbows tucked close to your body.

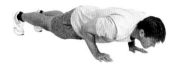

Easier option Perform the exercise on your knees, using your knees as the pivot point.

Dumbbell chest press (fly)

Muscles: Chest/shoulders (pectoral/deltoid) ✳ **Weight:** Dumbbells

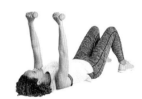

Start   Lie flat on the floor on your back, with your knees bent around 90 degrees, and feet flat on the floor. Hold a pair of dumbbells above your chest, about chest-width apart, with your arms straight and your palms facing forward.

Action   » Slowly lower the weights to the sides of your chest, until your upper arms touch the floor, keeping your elbows close to your body (not flared).

       » Pause, then push the weights back up to the starting position.

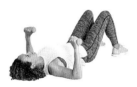

Tip You can begin by resting the dumbbells on your thighs, and do a gentle knee raise to help lift the dumbbells one at a time to the starting position.

Lying tricep extension

Muscles: Back upper arm (triceps) ✳ **Weight:** Dumbbells

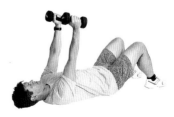

Start   Lie flat on the floor on your back, with your knees bent around 90 degrees, and feet flat on the floor. Hold a pair of dumbbells above your chest, with your arms straight and your palms facing each other.

Action   » Without moving your upper arms, bend your elbows and lower the dumbbells to the sides of your head, until your forearms dip below parallel to the floor.

       » Pause, then push the weights back up to the starting position.

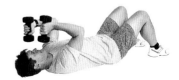

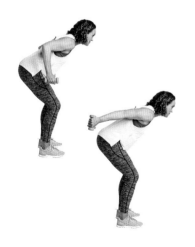

Tricep kickback

Muscles: Back upper arm (triceps) ✱ **Weight:** Dumbbells

Start   Stand upright with your knees bent slightly. Bend forward at the waist so you are leaning over your feet. Hold a dumbbell in each hand, palms facing each other, and bend your elbows to raise your upper arms so they are parallel to the floor. Your forearms should remain pointing down, and the front end of the dumbbells should be pointing forward. Keep your head up and facing forward.

Action » Keeping your torso stationary, your upper arms still and your elbows close to your torso, straighten your forearms behind you, until your entire arm is parallel to the floor and the front of the dumbbells point towards the floor.

» Pause, then slowly return the weights to the starting position.

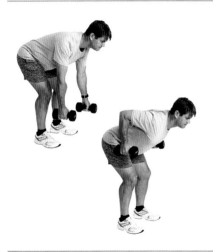

Bent-over row

Muscles: Back (latissimus dorsi, rhomboids) ✱ **Weight:** Dumbbells

Start   Stand with your feet shoulder-width apart, holding a dumbbell in each hand. Brace your core, push your hips back, bend your knees slightly and lower your torso until it's nearly parallel to the floor. Let the dumbbells hang at arms' length, with your palms facing each other. Engage your shoulder blades to keep your shoulders pulled back (i.e. don't hunch), and keep your head facing forward.

Action » Without moving your torso, and while keeping your chin and elbows tucked and back flat, 'row' the weights to the outsides of your ribcage as you squeeze your shoulder blades together.

» Pause, then slowly lower the weights to the starting position.

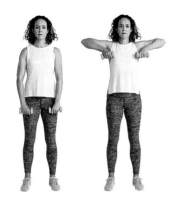

Upright row

Muscles: Upper back (trapezius) ✱ **Weight:** Dumbbells

Start   Stand tall with your arms down in front of you, and a dumbbell in each hand. Your palms should be facing your thighs.

Action » Keeping your torso stationary and your arms extended, lift the weights outwards and upwards, squeezing your shoulder blades until your arms are parallel to the floor.

» Pause, then slowly lower the weights to the starting position.

CORE (TRUNK)

Crunches

Muscles: Stomach (abdominals) * **Weight:** Body

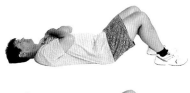
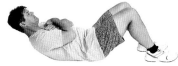

Start   Lie on your back with your legs bent and feet flat on the floor. Place your hands crossed in front of your chest.

Action » Imagine you're pulling your belly button back into your spine. Contract your abdominal muscles and raise your shoulder blades about 10 cm off the ground during the contraction.

      » Pause — you should feel a slight burn in your abdominals — then slowly return to the starting position.

Advanced To make it harder, hold something heavy on your chest, such as a textbook or weight.

Plank

Muscles: Stomach (abdominals) * **Weight:** Body

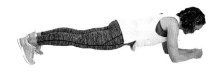

Start   Assume a push-up position, but with your weight on your forearms instead of your hands; your elbows should be directly beneath your shoulders, and your legs extended behind your body on your toes.

Action » Squeeze your glutes (buttocks) and brace your core to lock your body in a straight line from head to heels. Hold the position for 30–60 seconds (or as long as you can).

Easier option If the exercise is too difficult on your toes, you can drop your legs down to your knees as the pivot point.

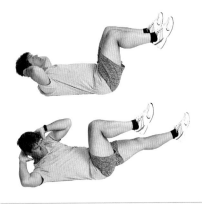

Bicycle

Muscles: Stomach (oblique abdominals) ✳ **Weight**: Body

Start Lie on your back with your hands behind your head, and elbows out to the side. Bend your knees at 90 degrees, so your lower legs are parallel to the floor. Lift your shoulder blades to the crunch position.

Action » With your knees in towards your chest, bring your left elbow towards your right knee as your left leg straightens, while crunching your stomach muscles. Continue alternating sides, as though you're pedalling on a bicycle, for 30–60 seconds.

Alternate limb raises

Muscles: Middle/lower back (erectors) ✳ **Weight**: Body

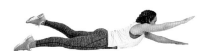

Start Lie on your stomach with your arms outstretched, palms facing the floor and legs straight out.

Action » Lift one arm and the opposing leg a few inches off the floor, keeping them straight, without rotating your shoulders, and keeping your head and torso still. Hold for a count of two, then lower your arm and leg back down.

» Now repeat with the opposite arm and leg.

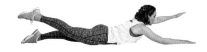

» A complete right- and left-side sequence equals one repetition. Alternate until the set is complete.

Advanced 1 Increase the length of time you hold the raised position.
Advanced 2 ('Superman') Raise both arms and legs simultaneously.

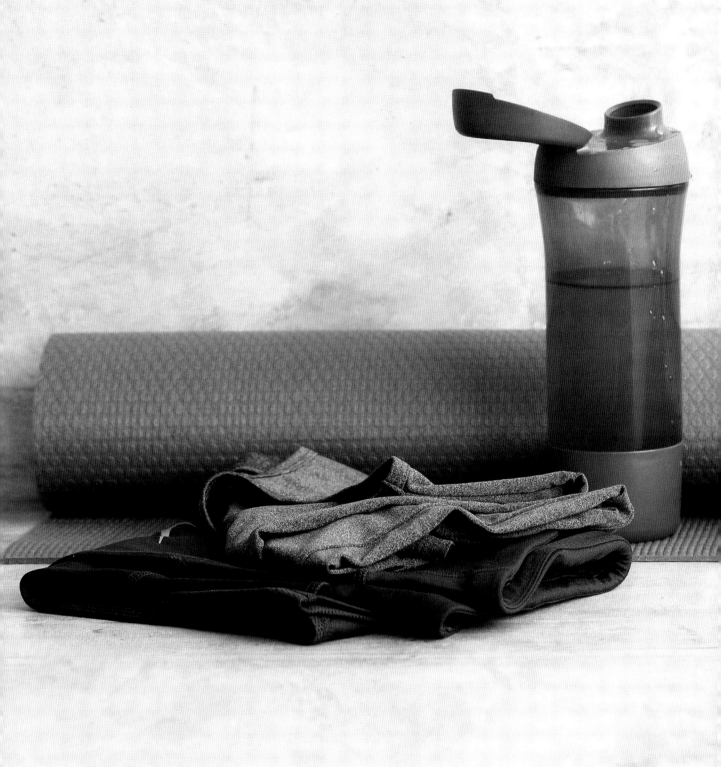

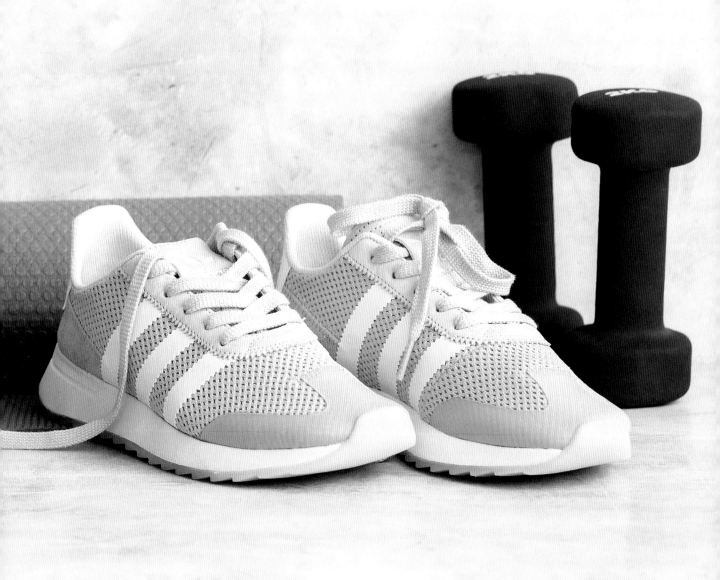

LOWER BODY

Dumbbell squat

Muscles: Bottom/thighs (glutes/quads) ＊ **Weight:** Body/dumbbells

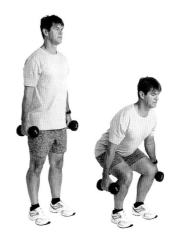

Start   Stand tall with your feet hip-width to shoulder-width apart, holding a pair of dumbbells at arms' length by your sides.

Action » Keeping your back flat and core braced, push your hips back, bend your knees and lower your body until your thighs are parallel to the floor. Make sure your heels do not rise off the floor. Avoid leaning so far forward that your knees go over the front of your toes.

     » Pause, then press through your heels to push yourself back up to the starting position.

Easier option Without holding the dumbbells, raise your arms in front of your body as you lower into the squat position.

Lunge

Muscles: Bottom/thighs (glutes/quads/hamstrings) ＊ **Weight:** Body/dumbbells

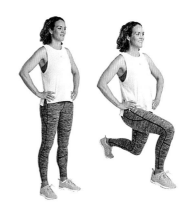

Start   Stand with your hands on your hips, and your feet hip-width apart.

Action » Step your right leg forward and slowly your lower body until your left (back) knee is close to touching the floor and is bent at least 90 degrees.

     » Pause, then slowly return to the starting position.

     » Repeat on the other side. A complete right- and left-side sequence equals one repetition.

Variation Try stepping back into the lunge.

Advanced Hold a dumbbell in each hand.

Calf raises

Muscles: Calf (gastrocnemius/soleus) ＊ **Weight:** Body/dumbbells

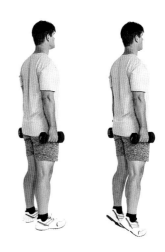

Start   Stand with your feet shoulder-width apart, supporting your weight on the balls of your feet. Hold a dumbbell in each hand by your side, with your palms facing your thighs.

Action » Raise your heels off the floor by contracting your calf muscles.

     » Pause, then slowly lower your heels back to the floor, to the starting position.

Easier option Perform the exercise without holding the dumbbells.

Advanced To increase the range of motion, start with your toes and the balls of your feet on a sturdy platform (such as a step), and your heels hanging off and touching the ground.

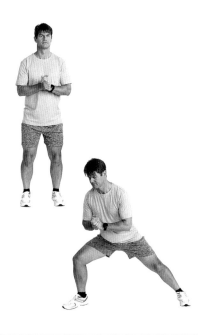

Side lunge

Muscles: Bottom/thighs (glutes/quads/hamstrings)
Weight: Body/dumbbell

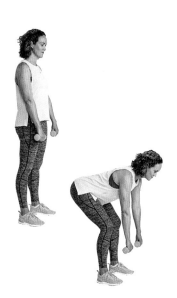

Start   Stand tall with your feet shoulder-width apart.

Action » Maintaining an upright position, step your right foot sideways, positioning your toes slightly outwards. Shift your body weight onto your right heel, then bend your right knee to slowly squat down until your right upper leg is parallel to the ground. Keep your chest high and your left knee extended to the side.

» Pause, then push back up from your right foot to the starting position.

» Repeat the movement with the left foot stepping sideways. A complete right- and left-side sequence equals one repetition.

Bodyweight version Clasp your hands together in front of your chest, with your elbows bent.

Dumbbell (advanced) version Hold a dumbbell between your hands (palms facing each other), in front of your chest, with your elbows bent.

Deadlifts

Muscles: Back/bottom/thighs (erectors/glutes/quads/hamstrings)
Weight: Body/dumbbells

Start   Stand tall with your arms pointing down in front of you, and a dumbbell in each hand. Your palms should be facing your thighs, and your weight should be on your heels.

Action » Keeping your body weight on your heels, and your arms down, bend at the hips to push your bottom backwards as far as possible, keeping your torso and stomach tight. Your knees should bend just a little, and you should keep your chest up and your back arched inwards.

» Pause, then slowly bring your hips forward to return to the starting position.

Easier option Perform the exercise without holding the dumbbells.

Single-leg deadlift

Muscles: Back/bottom/thighs (erectors/glutes/quads/hamstrings)
Weight: Body/dumbbells

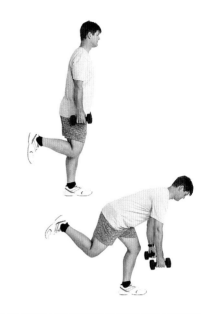

Start Stand tall with your arms pointing down in front of you, and a dumbbell in each hand. Your palms should be facing your thighs, and your weight should be on your heels.

Action » Lift your right leg slightly, and lower your arms and chest while raising your right leg behind your body, keeping your chest straight and stomach tight. Keep your left knee slightly bent and reach your arms as close to the floor as possible.

» Pause, then slowly return to the starting position by raising your chest while lowering the right leg.

» Repeat the movement by lifting the left leg. A complete right- and left-side sequence equals one repetition.

Easier option Perform the exercise without holding the dumbbells.

Shoulder bridge (glute bridge)

Muscles: Bottom/thighs/back/stomach (glutes/hamstrings/quads/erectors/abdominals) ✳ **Weight:** Body

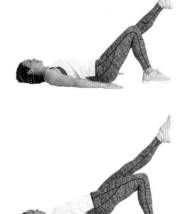

Start Lie on your back with your knees bent and feet hip-width apart. Place your arms at your side and lift up your spine and hips, so that only your head, feet, arms and shoulders are on the ground. Lift one leg upwards into a hip extension by squeezing your glutes, keeping your core tight. At the same time, press the heel of your other foot into the floor for more stability.

Action » Slowly bring your hips back down, then lift back up. Repeat for a specific number of repetitions, then bring your knee back in place and spine back to the floor.

» Repeat the movement on the other leg. A complete right- and left-side sequence equals one set.

Appendix

A simple equation to estimate your lean body mass

The amount of lean body (and fat) mass you have will vary according to your age, sex, height, weight and how physically active you are. If you don't have the equipment to assess your body composition, below is a simple calculator to help you estimate your lean body mass. It is important to remember these are predictive equations developed on population-specific data and, whilst they will provide you with a reasonable estimate, they will not necessarily give you the precise accurate measurement that could be provided with some of the other equipment tools described. Nevertheless, these equations can be useful for tracking your progress over time if you are trying to build muscle (and lean muscle tissue) and/or lose weight (body fat).

This equation calculates your percentage of lean body mass (which is the difference between total body weight and body fat weight expressed as a percentage), and is the reverse of your body fat percentage.

Formula for estimating your lean body mass

Men
[(0.407 x weight in kilograms) + (0.267 x height in centimetres) – 19.2] / weight in kilograms x 100

Women
[(0.252 x weight in kilograms) + (0.473 x height in centimetres) – 48.3] / weight in kilograms x 100

Note: there are a few different methods for calculating lean body mass. Here we've used the Boer Formula (Boer P. 'Estimated lean body mass as an index for normalization of body fluid volumes in man' Am J Physiol 1984; 247:F632–5).

How to calculate lean body mass, example 1

Susan is **160 centimetres tall** and weighs **57 kilograms**.

Her estimated lean body mass is therefore:
[(0.252 x weight in kilograms) + (0.473 x height in centimetres) – 48.3]
    / weight in kilograms x 100
[(0.252 x 57) + (0.473 x 160) – 48.3] / 57 x 100
[(14.364) + (75.68) – 48.3] / 57 x 100
(90.044 – 48.3) / 57 x 100
41.744 / 57 x 100
0.73 x 100
= 73%

**In this example, Susan has an estimated lean body mass of 73%.
In reverse this represents a body fat percentage of 27%.**

How to calculate lean body mass, example 2

Frank is **174 centimetres tall** and weighs **82 kilograms**.

His estimated lean body mass is therefore:
[(0.407 x 82) + (0.267 x 174) – 19.2] / 82 x 100
[(33.374) + (46.458) – 19.2] / 82 x 100
(79.832 – 19.2) / 82 x 100
60.632 / 82 x 100
0.74 x 100
= 74%

**In this example, Frank has an estimated lean body mass of 74%.
In reverse this represents a body fat percentage of 26%.**

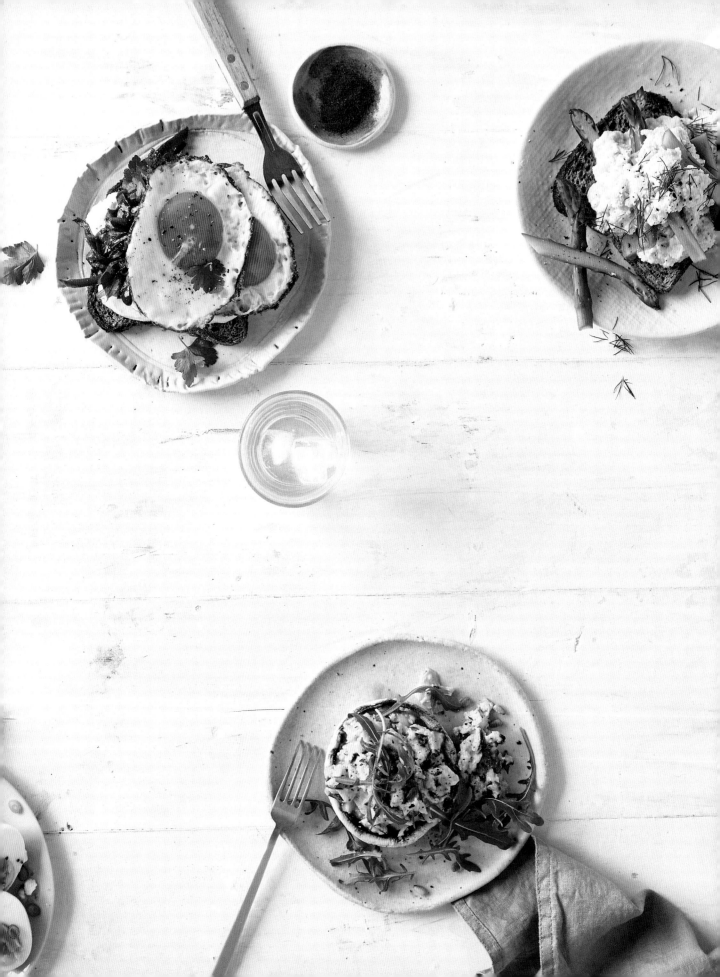

Lean body mass target guidelines

Generally, men and younger individuals tend to have a higher proportion of lean body mass than women or older individuals. For women, this is typically because they have more gender-specific body fat associated with them being able to bear children, and therefore tend to have less lean body mass than men.

On average, lean body mass ranges between 60–90% of body weight. Whilst it is not healthy to have a low lean body mass percentage, it also isn't healthy if your percentage of lean body mass is too high, as this means that you may not have enough body fat relative to lean mass. Body fat is essential for a range of normal functions. The table below provides a guide for percentage lean body mass and health*.

CLASSIFICATION OF BODY FAT LEVELS	AGE RANGE		
	MEN		
	20–39 years	**40–59 years**	**60–79 years**
Unhealthy (too much fat)	75% and lower lean body mass	72% and lower lean body mass	70% and lower lean body mass
Acceptable	76–80% lean body mass	73–78% lean body mass	71–75% lean body mass
Healthy	81–92% lean body mass	79–89% lean body mass	76–87% lean body mass
Unhealthy (too little fat)	More than 92% lean body mass	More than 89% lean body mass	More than 87% lean body mass
	WOMEN		
	20–39 years	**40–59 years**	**60–79 years**
Unhealthy (too much fat)	61% and lower lean body mass	60% and lower lean body mass	58% and lower lean body mass
Acceptable	62–67% lean body mass	61–66% lean body mass	59–64% lean body mass
Healthy	68–79% lean body mass	67–77% lean body mass	65–76% lean body mass
Unhealthy (too little fat)	More than 79% lean body mass	More than 77% lean body mass	More than 76% lean body mass

Adapted from Gallagher D, Heymsfield SB, Heo M, et al. 'Healthy percentage body fat ranges: an approach for developing guidelines based on body mass index.' Am J Clin Nutr. 2000; 72:694-701.

* The ranges described above are a rough estimate and should be used as a guide only. To determine the percentage of body lean and fat mass that is appropriate for your body we advise you consult your health professional. For example, a higher percentage of total lean mass and lower body fat may be more acceptable in certain sports where a low body fat is an advantage.

Recipe conversion chart

Measuring cups and spoons may vary slightly from one country to another, but the difference is generally not enough to affect a recipe. All cup and spoon measures are level.

One Australian metric measuring cup holds 250 ml (8 fl oz), one Australian tablespoon holds 20 ml (4 teaspoons) and one Australian metric teaspoon holds 5 ml. North America, New Zealand and the UK use a 15 ml (3-teaspoon) tablespoon.

LENGTH

METRIC	IMPERIAL
3 mm	⅛ inch
6 mm	¼ inch
1 cm	½ inch
2.5 cm	1 inch
5 cm	2 inches
18 cm	7 inches
20 cm	8 inches
23 cm	9 inches
25 cm	10 inches
30 cm	12 inches

LIQUID MEASURES

ONE AMERICAN PINT	ONE IMPERIAL PINT
500 ml (16 fl oz)	600 ml (20 fl oz)

CUP	METRIC	IMPERIAL
⅛ cup	30 ml	1 fl oz
¼ cup	60 ml	2 fl oz
⅓ cup	80 ml	2½ fl oz
½ cup	125 ml	4 fl oz
⅔ cup	160 ml	5 fl oz
¾ cup	180 ml	6 fl oz
1 cup	250 ml	8 fl oz
2 cups	500 ml	16 fl oz
2¼ cups	560 ml	20 fl oz
4 cups	1 litre	32 fl oz

DRY MEASURES

The most accurate way to measure dry ingredients is to weigh them. However, if using a cup, add the ingredient loosely to the cup and level with a knife; don't compact the ingredient unless the recipe requests 'firmly packed'.

METRIC	IMPERIAL
15 g	½ oz
30 g	1 oz
60 g	2 oz
125 g	4 oz (¼ lb)
185 g	6 oz
250 g	8 oz (½ lb)
375 g	12 oz (¾ lb)
500 g	16 oz (1 lb)
1 kg	32 oz (2 lb)

OVEN TEMPERATURES

CELSIUS	FAHRENHEIT	CELSIUS	GAS MARK
100°C	200°F	110°C	¼
120°C	250°F	130°C	½
150°C	300°F	140°C	1
160°C	325°F	150°C	2
180°C	350°F	170°C	3
200°C	400°F	180°C	4
220°C	425°F	190°C	5
		200°C	6
		220°C	7
		230°C	8
		240°C	9
		250°C	10

Notes

BAUER, J., et al. 2013. Evidence-based recommendations for optimal dietary protein intake in older people: a position paper from the PROT-AGE Study Group. *JAMA*, 14, 542–559.

BOSAEUS, I., et al. 2016. Nutrition and physical activity for the prevention and treatment of age-related sarcopenia. *Proc Nutr Soc*, 75, 174–180.

BOWEN, J., et al. 2008. Role of protein and carbohydrate sources on acute appetite responses in lean and overweight men. *Nutr Diet*, 65, S71–S78.

BOWEN, J., et al. 2006. Appetite regulatory hormone responses to various dietary proteins differ by body mass index status despite similar reductions in ad libitum energy intake. *J Clin Endocrinol Metab*, 91, 2913–2919.

BOWEN, J., et al. 2006. Energy Intake, Ghrelin, and Cholecystokinin after Different Carbohydrate and Protein Preloads in Overweight Men. *J Clin Endocrinol Metab*, 91, 1477–1483.

DEVRIES, M. C., et al. 2018. Protein leucine content is a determinant of shorter-and longer-term muscle protein synthetic responses at rest and following resistance exercise in healthy older women: a randomized, controlled trial. *Am J Clin Nutr*, 107, 217–226.

DHILLON, J., et al. 2016. The effects of increased protein intake on fullness: A meta-analysis and its limitations. *J Acad Nutr Diet*, 116, 968–983.

FOOD AND AGRICULTURE ORGANISATION OF THE UNITED NATIONS 2013. Dietary protein quality evaluation in human nutrition. Report of an FAO Expert Consultation. *FAO Food Nutr Paper*, 92, 1–66.

GOSBY, A., et al. 2014. Protein leverage and energy intake. *Obes Rev*, 15, 183–191.

HENDRIE, G., et al. 2016. Overconsumption of Energy and Excessive Discretionary Food Intake Inflates Dietary Greenhouse Gas Emissions in Australia. *Nutrients*, 8, 690.

KIM, I.-Y., et al. 2017. Update on maximal anabolic response to dietary protein. *Clin Nutr*, 37, 411–418.

LAYMAN, D. K., et al. 2015. Defining meal requirements for protein to optimize metabolic roles of amino acids. *Am J Clin Nutr*, 101, 1330S–1338S.

LEIDY, H. J., et al. 2015. The role of protein in weight loss and maintenance. *Am J Clin Nutr*, 101, 1320S–1329S.

LONGLAND, T. M., et al. 2016. Higher compared with lower dietary protein during an energy deficit combined with intense exercise promotes greater lean mass gain and fat mass loss: a randomized trial. *Am J Clin Nutr*, 103, 738–746.

MORTON, R. W., et al. 2018. A systematic review, meta-analysis and meta-regression of the effect of protein supplementation on resistance training-induced gains in muscle mass and strength in healthy adults. *Br J Sports Med*, 52, 376–384.

NATIONAL HEALTH AND MEDICAL RESEARCH COUNCIL 2013. Australian Dietary Guidelines. Canberra: National Health and Medical Research Council.

NATIONAL HEALTH AND MEDICAL RESEARCH COUNCIL 2006. Nutrient reference values for Australia and New Zealand. Canberra: National Health and Medical Research Council.

NOAKES, M. 2018. Protein Balance: New concepts for protein in weight management. Australia: CSIRO.

PHILLIPS, S. M., et al. 2016. Protein 'requirements' beyond the RDA: implications for optimizing health. *Appl Physiol Nutr Metab*, 41, 565–572.

QUATELA, A., et al. 2016. The energy content and composition of meals consumed after an overnight fast and their effects on diet induced thermogenesis: a systematic review, meta-analyses and meta-regressions. *Nutrients*, 8, 670.

SCHOENFELD, B. J., et al. 2018. How much protein can the body use in a single meal for muscle-building? Implications for daily protein distribution. *J Int Soc Sports Nutr*, 15, 10.

WEIGLE, D.S., et al. 2005. A high-protein diet induces sustained reductions in appetite, ad libitum caloric intake, and body weight despite compensatory changes in diurnal plasma leptin and ghrelin concentrations. *Am J Clin Nutr*. 82, 41–8

WITARD, O. C., et al. 2016. Growing older with health and vitality: a nexus of physical activity, exercise and nutrition. *Biogerontology*, 17, 529–546.

WOLFE, R. R., et al. 2018. Factors contributing to the selection of dietary protein food sources. *Clin Nutr*, 37, 130–138.

WYCHERLEY, T. P., et al. 2012. Effects of energy-restricted high-protein, low-fat compared with standard-protein, low-fat diets: a meta-analysis of randomized controlled trials. *Am J Clin Nutr*, 96, 1281–1298.

WYCHERLEY, T. P., et al. 2010. A high protein diet with resistance exercise training improves weight loss and body composition in overweight and obese patients with type 2 diabetes. *Diabetes Care*.

Index

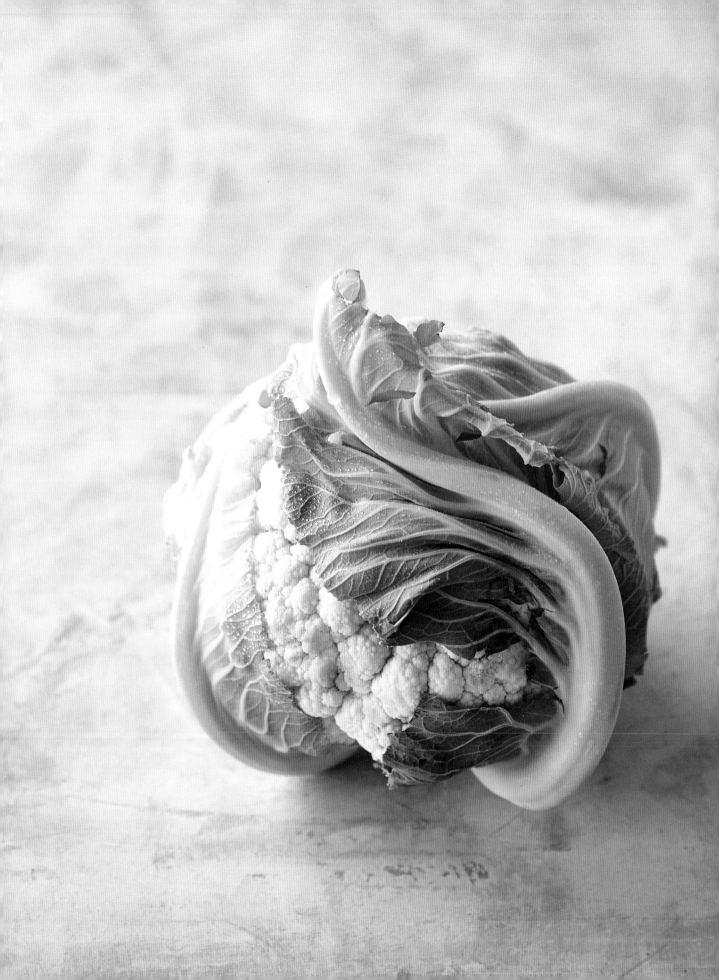

First published 2019 in Macmillan
by Pan Macmillan Australia Pty Limited
1 Market Street, Sydney, New South Wales
Australia 2000

A CIP catalogue record for this book is available from the
National Library of Australia: http://catalogue.nla.gov.au

Design by Sarah Odgers
Photography by Rob Palmer
Prop and food styling by Emma Knowles
Recipe development by Tracey Pattison
Food preparation by Peta Dent and Sarah-Jane Hallett
Editing by Katri Hilden and Rachel Carter
Colour + reproduction by Splitting Image Colour Studio
Printed in China by 1010 Printing International Limited

We advise that the information contained in this book
does not negate personal responsibility on the part of the
reader for their own health and safety. It is recommended
that individually tailored advice is sought from your
healthcare or medical professional. The publishers and
their respective employees, agents and authors are not
liable for injuries or damage occasioned to any person as
a result of reading or following the information contained
in this book.

10 9 8 7 6 5 4 3 2 1